The Deadly Dinner Party

The Deadly Dinner Party & Other Medical Detective Stories

~~~~~~~~

Jonathan A. Edlow, M.D.

~~~~~~~~

YALE UNIVERSITY PRESS
NEW HAVEN & LONDON

Published with assistance from the Louis Stern Memorial Fund

Designed by Nancy Ovedovitz and set in Janson Oldstyle type by
The Composing Room of Michigan, Inc. Printed in the United States
of America.

Library of Congress Cataloging-in-Publication Data
Edlow, Jonathan A.
The deadly dinner party : and other medical detective stories /
Jonathan A. Edlow.
    p.   cm.
Includes bibliographical references and index.
ISBN 978-0-300-12558-0 (alk. paper)
1. Medicine—Case studies.   I. Title.
[DNLM: 1. Diagnosis, Differential—Case Reports.   2. Disease—
etiology—Case Reports.   3. Epidemiologic Methods—Case Reports.
4. Infection—diagnosis—Case Reports.   5. Poisoning—diagnosis—
Case Reports.   WB 141 E23d 2009]
RC66.E35 2009
616.07′5—dc22   2009010830

A catalogue record for this book is available from the British Library.

This paper meets the requirements of ANSI/NISO Z39.48-1992
(Permanence of Paper).

10 9 8 7 6 5 4 3 2 1

I have been blessed to find the love of my life, Pamela. She encourages my writing because she knows I love it. She edits my work to make it less obtuse. She supports me when there is a deadline—which is most of the time! But most of all, she makes waking up each day exciting and gives me peace and hope.

Contents

Preface

~~~~~

When I was a teenager, my mother gave me a paperback book called *The Medical Detectives*, by Berton Roueché. These stories had all been previously published in an occasional series in the *New Yorker* called the Annals of Medicine. I had never heard of the *New Yorker* back then, and I had no particular desire to pursue a career in medicine. But I do remember devouring these stories one after another, and being sad when each one was over and sadder still when I had finished the book.

The volume was a collection of real-life medical mysteries—clusters of patients with odd symptoms, bizarre outbreaks of unusual diseases, and full-scale epidemics. The common thread was diagnosis, but not just any diagnosis. In each case, the solution proved tough to find. It was never a simple x-ray or routine blood test that made the final diagnosis, but doctors playing detective. Some physician or medical epidemiologist had to delve beneath the surface to find all the pieces and solve the puzzle. The first of these stories that I ever read was called "Eleven Blue Men." As it turns out, I was not the only person who found this story fascinating; the television series *House* used it for its pilot episode.

Another book that I read as a teenager was the *Complete Stories of Sherlock Holmes*. These yarns had the same effect on me, always making me wonder which facts would turn out to be clues and which were red herrings. I liked these stories and short novels so much that I reread the entire Sherlock Holmes canon as a college student.

Part of the appeal in both sets of stories was their length—not too short and not too long. As an adult, my attention span is not much longer than it was when I was a teenager, and I liked being able to read these tales in a single sitting. The second element they had in common was the simple pull of any detective story: figuring out "whodunit" and following, at least in retrospect, how the hero, whether an epidemiologist or Sherlock Holmes himself, solved the puzzle. Last, each of these miniature mysteries had all the elements of any good story—plot, character, and setting. The writing placed the reader in the midst of the investigation, just like Dr. Watson, the sidekick to Holmes.

Part of every doctor's and epidemiologist's job is to solve mysteries. Many are not so challenging. A patient consults a doctor because of fever and bloody diarrhea after eating undercooked hamburger. The doctor sends a stool culture and *E. coli* grows out. Case closed. Or a patient shovels heavy wet snow, develops chest pains, and comes to an emergency department. An electrocardiogram shows a heart attack. Another patient seeks medical advice in June for a low-grade fever and a large, unusual red rash over the abdomen at the site of a tick bite. It doesn't take a Sherlock Holmes to diagnose Lyme disease.

But sometimes, patients present problems that can be far more challenging. The clues lead to dead ends. The x-rays, blood tests, and CT scans are normal. Even smart doctors are unable to make a diagnosis. Or sometimes, they make a presumptive diagnosis, but the treatment fails. In these cases, the doctor becomes detective and the diagnosis can be as elusive as any criminal. Clues may not be so easy to find, sometimes because they are hiding out in the open, just as in Edgar Allan Poe's "The Purloined Letter." Sometimes doctors may call in the local public health epidemiologists to help with the problem. In other situations, if the scope of the outbreak overwhelms local resources, the Epidemiology Intelligence Service of the Centers for Disease Control and Prevention will be called in. Dr. Alexander Langmuir created this service in about 1950 when he began training a cadre of young physicians to become the country's medical sleuths.

The young men and women who work for this program today are available on a moment's notice, suitcases prepacked, to respond to any outbreak of disease or epidemic in the United States. They are famous for what Langmuir called "shoe-leather epidemiology." They solve cases the old-fashioned way, like the detectives in any good mystery story—by knocking on doors, interrogating witnesses, coming up with hypotheses, and then testing them.

With this in mind, as an adult I began collecting my own medical mysteries and was fortunate enough to have *Boston* magazine and *Ladies' Home Journal* publish some of them. I thank all the many individuals who made time to share parts of these stories with me.

People necessarily have an anthropocentric view of the world, but even though we may be at the top of the food chain, that doesn't mean we have dominion over the world or our environment. As Friedrich Nietzsche put it, "The human is by no means the crown of creation; every living kind stands beside it on the same level of perfection." In fact, we share our planet with an uncountable number of other species, each one scratching out its own ecological niche.

When humans fall ill to some virus or bacterium, it is simply the interplay between competitors in the same environment, each procreating and fulfilling its own biological destiny. Several of the stories here may be classified as "human meets pathogen." In "The Deadly Dinner Party," a notorious bug makes its mark and turns a suburban meal into a disaster that almost claims its host. This case shows how a microorganism can strike, not through a direct assault on human beings, but by a toxin that it elaborates. A tale like this provides an extraordinary lesson about the history of the relationship between humans and our cohabitants on the planet.

"Everywhere That Mary Went" exemplifies our struggle with another bacterium that has evolved such that *Homo sapiens* provides its only natural reservoir—hitchhiking, as it were, with our species. This is a story not only of an interesting outbreak of disease in the Catskills, but one about a malady that has had a major impact on human activities over centuries. "The Baby and the Bathwater," another case of infection, is a detective story par excellence. It shows how epidemiologists think and how shoe-leather epidemiology (not to mention hunches and an occasional bit of luck) plays into the solution of a mystery.

"Rubbed the Wrong Way" is a prime example of how the most mundane of human activities—personal hygiene—can lead to troublesome problems. Our microcosm becomes a bacteria's macrocosm, where several square feet of our body surface is their entire universe. Rounding out the first part of the book, "The Forbidden Fruit" illustrates not only the connection between bacteria and humans but the considerably more complex interplay of other animals, microorganisms, and people, sometimes with catastrophic results.

This last case introduces the importance of the world around us. Our relationship to nonliving parts of the environment is another category of exposure to illness. As fans of this genre will recognize, the title of the next story, "Two Ticks from Jersey," pays homage to Berton Roueché, whose "A Pig from Jersey," about trichinosis contracted from eating undercooked pork, was included in his original collection. In the tick story, we again see the ramifications of our life on a planet that we share with other creatures. Ticks have become increasingly important as vectors for a variety of diseases, mostly infectious. In this story, the lives of two little girls were in peril.

A large part of our lives is work, and work can sometimes be dangerous. In "An Airtight Case," a young executive was diagnosed with lung cancer. The odd thing was that his tumors seemed to wax and wane, and he was otherwise the picture of health. His physician was the detective who solved a mystery that baffled other doctors. "Monday Morning Fever" shows how a manufacturing process was central to the solution of a mini-epidemic in a small New England mill. This story is a classic example of how doctors see trees while epidemiologists see forests. Sometimes examining the commonalities in a group of cases helps to establish the diagnosis in an individual patient.

But we do not even need to leave the house for the environment to invade our space; it's everywhere. In "The Case of the Wide-Eyed Boy," we see how even a ten-year-old can be the victim, and how an emergency physician's sixth sense alerted him to the presence of an unusual problem that cracked the case.

We must also remember that there are really two "environments"—the internal and the external. The famous French physiologist Claude Bernard first introduced the term "internal milieu" to the scientific lexicon in 1865, when he wrote that the internal environment, in this case the inside of a cell, must be maintained within certain constant parameters for the cell to survive. But whether we mean an individual cell or an individual organism, this principle remains true. The interplay between internal and external environments is yet another category for diseases in humans.

In "A Study in Scarlet" (this time a nod to Sir Arthur Conan Doyle's story of the same title), an alert infectious diseases specialist at a medical conference suspects an unusual cause behind an outbreak of disease in a quaint New Hampshire hotel: once again, an epidemiologist's hunch plays a role in solving a colorful case. In another story, "The Case of the Overly Hot Honeymoon," the patient's brother (then a medical student) helped to unravel the mystery of why his sister could eat her football-playing husband under the table without gaining weight. This is a classic case of the internal milieu gone haywire.

In this day and age of food additives, irradiated fruits, genetic manipulation of crops, and fast food, eating healthily has become a near obsession for some. In "Feeling His Oats," a former advertising executive from Connecticut starts a health-food diet and almost eats himself to death by following the instructions in a best-selling diet book. "The Case of the Unhealthy Health Food" presents a similar theme. A suburban housewife suspected of having cancer undergoes numerous invasive tests and surgical procedures, but her diagnosis proves elusive. A curious medical student with time on his hands finds that the problem is not a cancer but, paradoxically, comes from a product that the patient is taking to feel better.

In "Little Luisa's Blinding Headache," a young girl nearly loses her vision from a health potion her grandmother had given to her with the best of intentions. The concoction contained substances that may be helpful at one dose but toxic at another. Finally, in "Too Much of a Good Thing," children in the Boston area get sick from something that belongs to a rite of childhood. When adults in the area also become ill, doctors begin to put the pieces of the puzzle together at a local educational conference.

The three categories of exposure to diseases are by no means simple and binary; they frequently overlap. Our world is a complex place; the interactions between host and environment (both external and internal) and pathogen can be equally complex. The lessons learned from these stories can help us negotiate this sometimes fragile relationship. My hope is that the reader will be able to profit from these stories through both their educational as well as their entertainment value.

PART ONE *Human Meets Pathogen*

~~~~~~~~~~~

The get-together began as an afterthought, recalls Pam Stogess, a forty-three-year-old city legislator from Kingston, New York, a town nestled between Catskill State Park and the Hudson River. "My husband, my daughter, and I were planning to go out for Mexican food. I asked our friend Steve Gelson to join us, but he invited us to his house to eat. Steve is a marvelous chef and had hosted a party the night before and had plenty of food left over. He said, 'nothing formal, don't get dressed up, just come over.' My husband and daughter were set on Mexican, but I went to Steve's. It was a totally last-minute affair."

Five other guests (the names of all persons in this story have been changed) attended the dinner party on Sunday, February 19, 1989: Miles Walsh, Steve's business partner in an ad agency; Arthur Landry, vice principal of the local high school; his wife, Barbara Landry, co-owner of their family travel agency; Janie, their thirteen-year-old daughter; and her friend Sara, also thirteen. The meal included a homemade cheese ball, salad, a pasta casserole with sausage, sweet-and-sour meatballs, garlic bread, and wine, followed by coffee and homemade fudge cake.

It turned out to be a memorable menu in more ways than one. "I doctored up the leftover pasta dish and made garlic bread out of pita slices," Gelson recalls. "It was a relaxing evening; we talked a lot of politics. Pam and I are active local Republicans, and Art, a Democrat, had just been told he would soon be appointed to a city commission."

"It was very informal," says Pam. "Steve arranged the food on the kitchen counter, and the adults ate in there. The girls took their plates into the living room and watched videos. We had a grand time, but it was a school night, so by 10 PM, we finished our coffee and the party was over."

By Tuesday morning, Pam knew something was wrong. "I was working in the kitchen; I looked up at something, and my eyes wouldn't work right. I thought maybe I'd put my contact lenses in backwards, so I went into the bathroom, cleaned and checked them, and put them back on. But things still weren't right; it was like I was looking at my nose cross-eyed. I figured I had the flu.

"I phoned Steve's office, because as trustees of the Ulster County YWCA, we had a noon meeting. His secretary told me he was home sick, and when I called him, his speech was slurred, and he complained of nausea. He said he wouldn't be coming to the meeting. I said that I'd speak with him at dinner time and to let me know what he wanted and that I'd make it and bring it over to him.

"By that evening [Tuesday]," Pam continues, "my eyes were worse and my speech had also become slurred. I was having trouble talking and remember having to form the words to get them out. I called Steve again that evening and he could hardly speak. Then the idea occurred to me that Steve and I had the same bug."

Still, Pam isn't the panicky type and still wasn't particularly concerned about her own health. She assumed that she probably just had a virus that would eventually run its course.

"Wednesday morning, I started to drive to do some errands, but as I pulled out of the driveway, the street didn't look wide enough for the car, so my husband drove me. When I went to sign a check, I couldn't find the right line. I was trying to hold some toothpicks but kept dropping them. It was odd. I was having perceptual problems and it gave me a whole new perspective on how handicapped people must have to deal with the world."

By Thursday morning, Pam felt so feeble "that it was all I could do to walk, my legs were so weak. By now I was getting nervous, and I'm not the nervous type. My husband and I own a funeral home, and the prospect of death doesn't frighten me. I remember telling my husband, 'I think I've had a stroke,'" Pam recalls. "I felt intoxicated and totally out of touch perceptually. I telephoned Steve's house and there was no answer. I called his secretary, who told me he'd gone to Kingston Hospital. That's when I thought, 'My God, maybe someone else has it.' I called Art Landry's house.

"Janie picked up and said her dad couldn't come to the phone; he was sick and couldn't speak. Janie and Barbara were fine, though. By now, I was having difficulty swallowing, chewing, or even moving my tongue. I called Dr. Mauceri, Steve's doctor, and told him about Art and me. He said we should both come to the emergency department at Kingston City Hospital [where Steve was being evaluated] for tests."

Dr. Mauceri had already paid Steve two house calls. Mauceri was not only Gelson's doctor but also a friend; in fact, he had been a guest at the first dinner party on Saturday night. He saw Steve at home on Wednesday and was somewhat concerned, but when he saw him again on Thursday, at about 2 PM, he sent Gelson straight to the hospital. "I remember he took my portable phone," said Steve, "and called a neurologist, Dr. Pickard, on the telephone. He said, 'I've got a patient I'd like you to see today. I'm concerned he could have Guillain-Barré syndrome.'"

By four o'clock that afternoon, the consulting neurologist, Dr. Leonard Pickard, was evaluating Steve Gelson in the emergency department. Pickard at this point was still unaware that Art and Pam were also ill. When he finished examining Steve, he was both puzzled and worried. Two major possibilities occurred to him—myasthenia gravis and Guillain-Barré syndrome, both potentially fatal neurological disorders. "But Steve's symptoms didn't quite fit with either diagnosis," Pickard recalls, "and there was one other possibility that Dr. Mauceri and I discussed."

Pam Stogess remembers, "Shortly after 4 PM, Art and I joined Steve at the emergency room, and we must have been quite a sight. Steve's head hung limp to one side. His eyelids drooped shut so that when he spoke, he had to pry them open with his fingers. Art, a community leader, looked like a drunken bum. He hadn't shaved for a couple of days, and he wore a baseball cap cocked to one side."

"After I examined Mr. Gelson," recalls Dr. Pickard, "his father told me about Pam Stogess and Art Landry. The clustering of cases was what clinched it. Even though I'd never seen a case, I knew they had botulism."

Botulism, which derives from *botulus*, the Latin word for sausage, is a rare but often fatal form of food poisoning caused by the bacterium *Clostridium botulinum*. According to Dr. A. Barnett Christie's eminently readable textbook on epidemiology and infectious diseases, the history of the word "botulism" and the discovery of the causative organism dates back more than two hundred years. Christie wrote, "The term was first used in the last years of the eighteenth century following an outbreak of the disease in Wildbad, in Southern Germany, in 1793: a large sausage had been shared by thirteen people, all of whom became ill and six of whom died."

Much of what is currently known about the clinical effects of botulism was catalogued by a young district medical officer in the duchy of Württemberg named Dr. Justinus Kerner. At the beginning of the nineteenth century in the area surrounding Stuttgart, the medical administration of the dukedom noticed an increase in cases of fatal food poisoning, which they ascribed to the general decline in hygienic measures for food production that resulted from the poverty caused by the devastating Napoleonic wars. In July 1802, the government in Stuttgart issued a public notice and warning about the "harmful consumption of smoked blood sausages."

Kerner, who also developed a lasting reputation as a Romantic poet, began publishing his findings in 1817. By 1820, he had written a monograph that included data from seventy-six patients he had seen with "sausage poisoning," as it was referred to at the time. Kerner performed animal experiments and did many autopsies on patients who had died from botulism. By the mid-1820s, he had established most of what we currently know to be true. He wrote, "The tear fluid disappears, the gullet becomes a dead and motionless tube. . . . No saliva is secreted. No drop of wetness is felt in the mouth, no tear is secreted anymore."

Using various extracts that he made from the sausages, Kerner experimented on cats, rabbits, birds, snails, insects, and frogs. He was able to produce all the typical symptoms—dilated pupil, droopy eyelids, vomiting, problems with swallowing, and respiratory failure—in these animals. But Kerner went even further. Like many physicians of his time, he experimented on himself. After taking very diluted extracts from the sausage, he wrote, "some drops of the acid brought onto the tongue [produced] great drying out of the palate and the pharynx." When the university professor who had been his instructor discovered that Kerner was poisoning himself in the name of research, he wisely forbade future self-experimentation.

Although Kerner tried in vain to produce the toxin, he did uncover the three major principles about sausage poisoning: he learned that the toxin is created in the bad sausage when it is stored in an oxygen-free state; that the toxin acted on both the motor and autonomic portions of the nervous system; and that the toxin was extremely potent and could lead to symptoms in very small doses. Most remarkably, Kerner speculated in his 1820 report that certain diseases that are caused by a "hyperstimulated" or "hyperexcited" nervous system might in fact be treated by the toxin.

It was not until 1870 that the word "botulism" was formally coined by another German physician. It took nearly thirty more years for the causative organism to be defined, in part because the necessary tools of bacteriology were still in their infancy during the late nineteenth century.

Finding the organism that was actually causing botulism is a story in itself. It starts in the tiny village of Ellezelles, Belgium. Thirty-four individuals attended a funeral on a cold day in December 1895. The food served for the occasion included both smoked and pickled ham. The latter had been pickled within twenty-four hours of slaughter and kept in brine for eleven days before it was consumed. It didn't look right and it didn't smell right, but that did not seem to have dampened the enthusiasm with which it was eaten by the guests and members of the village band, who apparently were playing both for the funeral as well as a local festival. The first victims fell ill in less than twenty-four hours, and in all, twenty-three people became sick. Three died, and ten nearly died. Some who had eaten smaller amounts had a mild illness, and a few, who had eaten only fat or very small pieces of the meat, had no symptoms at all.

Dr. Emile Pierre van Ermengem, who had studied under the great German pathologist Robert Koch, investigated. He found a large anaerobic (grows in the absence of oxygen) bacillus (long bacterium) in the ham that had been served at the funeral and in the tissues of some of the victims as well. From these samples, he grew the bacteria in the laboratory. Finally, when he fed cats food laced with the organism, they developed paralysis. Dr. Ermengem had finally found the cause. He published his findings in a German microbiology journal. This was the first recorded isolation of *Clostridium botulinum*. Nine years later, in 1904, an outbreak of botulism from canned white beans surprised researchers, for it had been thought that only meat or fish could lead to the disease.

Over succeeding decades, researchers worked out additional details that built on the early pioneers' theories. The active bacterium, *C. botulinum*, has a biological peculiarity in that it grows only in the absence of oxygen. The organism has an inactive stage called a spore. The spores can live indefinitely, even in extreme cold or heat; they remain active even after being boiled for hours. Under anaerobic conditions, the spores germinate into the active bacterium, and then the bacteria produce the toxin, one of the most deadly known. Somewhat unbelievably, in 1964 it was estimated that fourteen ounces of botulism toxin could kill the entire population of the world. Kerner was quite fortunate with his forays in self-experimentation, because even so much as a nibble of tainted food can be fatal.

In one small outbreak, in Loch Maree, Scotland, in 1923, eight members of a fishing party lunched on duck paté sandwiches; within a week, all eight were dead. Botulism toxin, a relatively small molecule, affects the nervous system by rapidly and tightly binding to the area where the nerve transmits its impulse to the muscle. Normally, the transmission of this impulse from the nerve to a muscle is mediated by the release of a chemical neurotransmitter, acetylcholine. The acetylcholine then binds to the muscle, causing it to contract. If insufficient acetylcholine binds to the muscle side of the connection, the muscle will not fire. If the diaphragm, the muscle that controls breathing, is affected, one can no longer breathe and will die unless emergency treatment is begun.

There are at least seven types of *C. botulinum*—somewhat unimaginatively labeled A through G—but types A, B, and E cause most disease in humans. The bacteria, and its spores, are everywhere, yet botulism is quite rare. In part this is because, although the spores are quite hardy, the toxin is quite frail. Even though heating does not destroy the spores, it routinely destroys the toxin, an Achilles heel that the prudent cook must exploit to avoid the dreaded disease. Contaminated food does not always show signs (such as blown cans or putrid smells) of being contaminated.

Consider the case of a twenty-two-year-old man from Orange County,

California. He awoke one morning at 2 AM, vomiting, with blurred vision and a "thick tongue." Within hours, he was completely paralyzed and he had stopped breathing. He was placed on a ventilator for respiratory support. About forty hours before the onset of his symptoms, he had eaten some stew that his roommate had prepared from fresh ingredients (meat, carrots, and potatoes). The roommate had eaten the same stew while it was still hot, but the other man had tasted it at room temperature, sixteen hours later. The heat-resistant spores had survived the first cooking. Any toxin that was in the stew would have been deactivated by the heating, which is why the roommate remained well. While the food was cooling on the stovetop, however, the spores, deep in the stew (and therefore in an anaerobic environment) germinated into *C. botulinum* bacteria. When the temperature became cool enough, the live bacteria began making toxin, which caused the young man to fall dangerously ill.

Cooking food to a high enough temperature just before it is eaten will reliably prevent the disease. According to Christie's textbook: "It is clear that any food may cause botulism if it is contaminated with the organism and is first given inadequate heat treatment, then stored for some time, and finally eaten without further cooking. This last point is important, for it will be remembered that botulinum toxin is easily destroyed by heat, and if only home-canned food were re-cooked before being eaten, most of the deaths caused by home-canned food could be avoided."

Botulism usually develops when a person eats improperly processed food. Outbreaks have been attributed to bottled mushrooms, roasted eggplant in oil, baked potatoes, stews, soups, sautéed onions, carrot juice, home-canned fruits and vegetables, chili, meat, and fish. In one sad cluster in 1975, an elderly woman canned some mushrooms, ate some of them, and promptly died. After the funeral, her daughter and daughter-in-law ate some more of the canned mushrooms and they both developed botulism. Type B *C. botulinum* was isolated from the mushrooms as well as the gastrointestinal tracts of all three women.

In 2002, fourteen Alaskans dined on the meat from a beached whale. Eight developed botulism, and two would have died without ICU-level care. Native Alaskans are particularly at risk because they eat seal and whale meat, and their most common food preparation practice is to ferment the flesh. In this process, the fresh meat is allowed to putrefy for one to two weeks in either a pit in the ground or a closed or airtight container. This anaerobic environment is ideal for the formation of botulism toxin.

One large outbreak was traced to commercially canned soup. On a hot day in mid-June 1971, a sixty-one-year-old banker and his wife from Bedford Village, New York, cooled off with some chilled vichyssoise. They didn't eat the whole bowl because it had an odd taste, but they ate enough. By the next morning, the man had double vision, followed by weakness of his entire body. Twenty-four hours later, he was dead. Only after his wife developed similar symptoms did the doctors suspect botulism. On July 2, the Food and Drug Administration (FDA) released a public warning after learning about the death, and the soup company, Bon Vivant of Newark, New Jersey, launched a recall of the 6,444 cans of vichyssoise that came from the same batch.

Bon Vivant manufactured 4 million cans of soup per year, so finding and retrieving these particular cans was no small feat. Five cans of the vichyssoise were found to be contaminated with the botulinum toxin, and cans from the company's other products also showed signs of improper handling. Therefore the FDA extended the recall to include all Bon Vivant products, and shut down the company's plant in Newark just five days after the original warning. By the end of the summer, the company had filed for bankruptcy.

Alaskan salmon is another source of at least two instances of botulism linked to commercially canned food. One of the most recent occurrences from a commercially prepared product was the Castleberry canned chili outbreak that erupted during the summer of 2007. Two patients from Texas and two others from Indiana became severely ill. The first two cases were a brother and sister from Lubbock, Texas. Both ate some canned chili made by the Castleberry Company, based in Atlanta, Georgia. Both required long hospitalizations; the sister was on a ventilator for more than a month. What is noteworthy in these cases is how widely scattered geographically the victims can be.

In another unusual outbreak, in 1979 in Nairobi, Kenya, botulism resulted from people eating white ants, which are nutritious even if unappetizing to some. The ants were caught in Kakamega, three hundred miles from Nairobi. People who ate fresh ants there remained well. But others placed the ants in sealed plastic bags and brought them to Nairobi three days later. By then enough time had elapsed in this oxygen-free environment so that the Clostridia spores that were present germinated and began producing toxin. Five of the six people who ate the transported white ants died from botulism. Foods that are entirely unprocessed and uncooked do not lead to botulism, as long as they are eaten fresh (because the spores themselves do not cause the disease); some kind of storage or processing is required for the toxin to form.

Two other forms of this disease should be mentioned—wound botulism and infant botulism. In wound botulism, spores in a closed contaminated wound can germinate into the bacteria that then form toxin, which is released into the circulation. This same mechanism has been reported in intravenous drug users. Infant botulism, a newcomer to the botulism family, was recognized only in 1976. In this form of the disease, infants between one and thirty-eight weeks old ingest foods that contain the spores, which germinate in the intestine, where they then form toxin, which is absorbed into the baby's bloodstream. The baby develops constipation, then altered sucking, swallowing, and crying and finally becomes "floppy." Some cases of sudden infant death syndrome may be due to botulism. Because honey contains *C. botulinum* spores and has been associated with clinical cases of infant botulism, pediatricians advise that children less than a year old not be fed honey.

There is even one other form of botulism. Precisely as Justinus Kerner predicted, botulinum toxin is now used therapeutically in an odd assortment of syndromes of hyperactive muscle tone—various dystonias, and spasm of the eyelids. More recently, and very commonly, the toxin is used for cosmetic reasons. Marketed as Botox, it temporarily paralyzes the facial muscles, which reduces wrinkles. In 2006, a thirty-four-year-old woman received a Botox injection from a friend who was an unlicensed physician. The product was research grade, but not pharmaceutical grade. Two days after the injection, she developed double vision, problems swallowing, and weakness. By the time she called an ambulance, her breathing was failing. She was placed on a ventilator and treated with antitoxin. However, her case progressed so rapidly to complete paralysis that it was three weeks before she could shrug her shoulders or move her eyes, and five weeks before she could speak. After a nearly four-month hospital stay, she was discharged to a rehabilitation facility.

In the standard food-borne botulism, symptoms typically begin within thirty-six hours after ingestion of the toxin, and include dry mouth and difficulty talking and swallowing. Patients frequently have double vision from problems with the muscles that move the eyes up and down and from side to side. Blurred vision also occurs in the majority of cases, perhaps from the droopy eyelids, or ptosis, as physicians call it. Fatigue is profound. In half of the instances, nausea and vomiting never occur, so many patients do not suspect a food-related illness. Fever is absent, and the victims remain mentally intact.

As recently as thirty years ago, as many as half of all botulism cases proved fatal. Improvements in intensive care, use of ventilators for respiratory failure, and the development of an antitoxin have dramatically lowered that dismal statistic. Of course the benefit of those improvements is all predicated on making an accurate diagnosis. Today severely afflicted patients can be placed on sophisticated ventilators for weeks if necessary, until the poison's deadly grip on the diaphragm has relaxed. The antitoxin is horse serum, prepared by immunizing horses with injections of botulism toxin, then extracting the horse's antibody-rich blood serum and giving it to patients. Because the antitoxin is a horse-serum product, patients may develop allergic side effects from the foreign protein, sometimes severe ones.

Because of these side effects, doctors like to be sure of the diagnosis before administering a therapy so potentially toxic. On the other hand, because the antitoxin must be delivered as rapidly as possible, they often must give the treatment based on a presumptive diagnosis.

Pam Stogess and Art Landry's doctors wanted to try to exclude Guillain-Barré syndrome, another cause of paralysis that can also affect a patient's ability to breathe, so they performed spinal taps on these dinner-party guests. If they had Guillain-Barré, the protein levels in the spinal fluid should be high.

They weren't.

Dr. Pickard phoned the federal Centers for Disease Control and Prevention (CDC) as soon as he thought that the diagnosis of botulism was likely. His next call was to the state health officials. At 5 PM on Thursday, Perry Smith of the New York State Department of Health in Albany took Pickard's call. Alarmed, he immediately informed his director, Dale Morse.

Morse recalls, "Dr. Smith received the call and we each got on the phone. Stan Kondracki [an epidemiologist] was about to step on the elevator to leave for the day, and I motioned for him to come back. I had him begin working on mobilizing the antitoxin from New York City, while Perry was still on the line with Dr. Pickard. Meanwhile, I began talking with the Ulster County officials. We did a lot of work in a very short period of time. We also had to notify the state lab to be prepared to receive specimens used to confirm the diagnosis."

In the command post hastily assembled to deal with the emerging epidemic, Kondracki quickly arranged for release of the antitoxin. The CDC headquarters, in Atlanta, maintains stockpiles at strategic locations across the country and keeps a phone line available to physicians twenty-four hours per day, seven days per week. The nearest antitoxin was at the quarantine station at John F. Kennedy Airport in New York City, about 115 miles away.

Until this point, Pam Stogess hadn't been particularly frightened about the disease. But when she heard about the cure, she finally understood that her life was in danger. "The doctors explained that there are sometimes serious side effects to the antitoxin, including fatal allergic reactions. That's when I realized how grave the situation was."

In the meantime, Ulster County health inspectors Brian Devine and Kevin DuMond had arrived at the Kingston hospital. "I got a call at home," remembers Devine, "from my director, who requested that I initiate an investigation of a possible botulism outbreak. We arrived at the hospital at around 6:15 PM. After interviewing the patients, we questioned the people who attended the dinner party who had not fallen ill, to determine who had eaten which foods." They tallied up just who had eaten what, and based on this information the inspectors singled out two likely culprits—the garlic bread and the cheese ball. Since all seven diners had eaten the casserole, the sausage (ironically, given the origin of the word "botulism") was an unlikely source of the toxin. Steve Gelson,

Pam Stogess, and Art Landry had all eaten the garlic bread, but so had Barbara Landry.

The CDC had already notified Pickard that a garlic-in-oil preparation had been responsible for a 1985 outbreak in Vancouver, Canada. That incident came to light when two teenage sisters and their mother, who had traveled from Vancouver to Montreal, developed visual problems, difficulty swallowing, and weakness. Botulism was diagnosed. They had eaten at a family-style restaurant back in Vancouver. When this was publicized, many more cases were identified. Ultimately this outbreak became one of the largest ever in North America, affecting thirty-six people from three countries, including several areas of the United States and eight Canadian provinces. The source turned out to be garlic packed in oil, which was supposed to be kept refrigerated but had not been.

When a cluster of typical cases occurs, little else but botulism can explain it; however, nature is not always that accommodating to the diagnostician. One of the most interesting aspects of the Vancouver outbreak was the long list of incorrect diagnoses that these patients were given before the botulism was identified in the three women. Seven had been diagnosed with myasthenia gravis, and four each with viral syndromes and psychiatric disturbances. Three each were diagnosed with stroke and Guillain-Barré syndrome, and many others with a myriad of other conditions (including overexertion). Only the twin sisters and their mother, representing less than 10 percent of the victims, were correctly diagnosed on the first visit to a physician. Most doctors will never see even a single case of botulism in their entire professional careers, which makes Dr. Pickard's rapid diagnosis all the more impressive.

Following up on the CDC's lead about the garlic and oil, Devine found an eight-ounce jar of Colavita minced garlic packed in extra virgin olive oil. "We arrived at Gelson's house at about 10 PM and took samples of the garlic in oil, the cheese, and the sausage used in the pasta casserole. We sent these to the state lab in Albany for testing." The garlic had been packed in oil, shielding it from oxygen, and it was not acidified with preservatives. Also, it had been stored at room temperature. This combination provided a near perfect environment for the spores to germinate into bacteria, which could then produce the toxin in the jar. On Sunday, the evening of the get-together, Steve prepared the garlic bread by slicing pita pockets into eighths, brushing on margarine, garlic, and oil, and then passing them briefly under the broiler—too briefly, as it turned out, to neutralize the toxin. Food must be heated to at least 176 degrees Fahrenheit for fifteen minutes to destroy the botulism toxin.

Before sending the samples to the lab in Albany, Devine carefully wrapped and labeled each one—an important precaution, since laboratory workers have gotten botulism by inhaling the toxin from improperly prepared samples. At the makeshift command post, Stan Kondracki was working on getting the antitoxin to the patients, but time and weather were working against him. "The CDC officials released the antitoxin quickly. But it was around rush hour, and the bridges around New York City were backed up, so sending it by ground would take too long. We also missed the last commercial flight out. So I called the state police. Although the weather was not favorable, the police dispatched a helicopter to JFK."

The pilot, Technical Sergeant John Ludweig, remembers, "I got a call from Captain [Lou] Grosso at approximately 6 PM. He told me there was some kind of serious problem in Kingston. I was at Stewart Airport and needed to pick something up from JFK and take it to Kingston. It was pretty windy on the ground." Ludweig flew to JFK, picked up the parcel, lifted off from the tarmac, dipped the helicopter's nose to the west, and pushed forward into the stiff headwind. After a brief but bumpy flight, he touched down on the landing pad at Kingston's Benedictine Hospital. Local police officers in squad cars met him there. With lights and sirens, the police relayed the serum across town to Kingston Hospital, where all three patients had been admitted to the intensive care unit.

Steve Gelson's condition was deteriorating.

The decision to administer antitoxin is not one that is made lightly. About 20 percent of patients receiving the treatment develop side effects. Because the attending physicians almost never know for sure which type of botulism the patient has at this early stage, they administer a "trivalent" product that protects against all three of the common strains—A, B, and E. For severely afflicted patients, like Gelson, the risk-benefit ratio clearly favors using the medication. But Pam Stogess wasn't so sure.

"We were told there was an antitoxin, but that it had some very serious possible side effects, even the possibility of dying from it. I was frightened by this and decided to wait until the next morning to decide. By Friday morning, I couldn't even pick up my toothbrush, and I decided to get the antitoxin. I got headaches and a rash that lasted two to three weeks. My whole body turned purple and my face swelled up, and then all of it gradually subsided, but I feel very fortunate to have recovered."

On Friday morning, five days after the dinner get-together, Brian Devine shipped the samples he had taken from Gelson's kitchen to the state lab in Albany for testing. By the next day, the state lab had preliminary results suggesting that this was indeed botulism; two days later the lab confirmed that the garlic in oil contained type A botulism toxin, the same type that was later isolated from the patients.

On March 1, 1989, the New York State Health Department issued a public advisory to inform people that they should discard any jars of the Colavita-brand garlic in oil. The following day, the FDA also issued a warning on the product. The manufacturer, the Colavita Pasta and Olive Oil Company of Newark, New Jersey, voluntarily recalled the product. In all, three hundred cases of four-, eight-, and thirty-two-ounce jars had been produced. Steve Gelson, Art Landry, and Pam Stogess later filed a lawsuit against the manufacturer, the distributor, and their local retailer of the product.

Inspector Devine tried to track the particular jar that Gelson used. Gelson had received the jar of garlic in oil in a Christmas gift basket, along with other Colavita products. The health inspector's report is ambiguous as to whether Gelson had stored the jar at room temperature or refrigerated it before opening it for the first time. After the first use, like most conscientious cooks, Gelson always kept it refrigerated. But like most people, he didn't realize that refrigeration would not inactivate any preformed toxin. Garlic comes from the soil, which can contain botulism spores. In the oil, an oxygen-free environment, the spores can germinate and lead to toxin formation. Also, the product was not acidified at the factory with citric or phosphoric acid, a process that would have diminished the likelihood of toxin formation.

Devine learned that Gelson had used the jar of Colavita garlic in oil three times. The first time was a few months earlier, when he added the garlic to a heated chicken dish. The second occasion was when he put it in the pasta casserole he served on Saturday night (the one that Dr. Mauceri had attended, the night before the small impromptu get-together). None of the guests from the Saturday-night affair got sick because the dish had been served piping hot. The third time was on the fateful Sunday-night dinner party.

Ultimately, all three victims recovered, although it took several months before they were fully recuperated, and to some extent none of them felt truly normal for years afterward. During the 1950s and 1960s, the mortality rate in cases of botulism was approximately 50 percent. In the 1990s, that rate fell to 5–10 percent, thanks to development of the antitoxin and modern ICU-level care—but it is still a number that is alarmingly high if you are one of those affected or know someone who is.

And the guests know that things might have turned out much worse. Most of the people at Steve Gelson's house that night never ate any of the garlic bread, as Pam explains. "We didn't have room for all the food on the counter, so Steve left the garlic bread on the oven behind his seat. The girls didn't see it when they filled their plates before retreating to the living room. Halfway through the meal, Steve remembered the garlic bread and offered it around. Miles declined. Art, Barbara, and I each took only one small chip. Steve ate five or six pieces during the rest of the evening." Barbara Landry was the one person who ate the garlic bread but did not get sick, either because her particular piece contained very little garlic or because she didn't eat as large a piece as the others.

The host, Steve Gelson, ate the most garlic bread, and therefore ingested the largest amount of the toxin. Doctors at the hospital had to put him on a mechanical ventilator to restore his breathing, inserting a plastic tube into his trachea to deliver oxygen to his lungs. "I can still feel that tube going down my throat," he recalls, years later, "and how for the first 15–20 seconds on the ventilator, you feel like you can't breathe. I was sedated but awake, and it was very panicky. I was on the ventilator for about two weeks and in the intensive care unit for about five weeks." He added ruefully, "I only used two teaspoons of garlic in oil for the bread. I never understood how toxic such a tiny amount of a substance can be."

~~~~~~~~~~~~~~~~

Roy Harvey, a postal clerk from Summerton, New York, married Rita Osborn, both in their early forties, on June 3, 1989 (their names and the town's name are fictional). Harvey, who doubles as an assistant chief of the local fire department, knew that the New York State Association of Fire Chiefs' convention was going to be held June 11–14, in the Catskills, and he had planned to attend. With a busy work schedule, finding time for their honeymoon was difficult, but the Catskill Mountains are beautiful that time of year. "So we figured we'd make that our honeymoon too," Harvey recalls. "We had a wonderful time, and I left feeling fine." But that feeling of well-being was not to last.

"We were at our camp at Alexandra Bay, on the St. Lawrence River, for July Fourth weekend and I really began to feel sick—like I was coming down with the flu: fevers, headaches. I swallowed aspirins by the ton, but they didn't help. I felt bad enough so that on Monday, July 3, when my temperature hit 104 degrees, I took myself to the local hospital." The doctors there examined him and agreed with the self-diagnosis of the flu. But the next day, Roy felt even worse. "The weather was really hot, but I was so chilly and freezing that I needed blankets. And my headache was blinding; I didn't even want to open my eyes.

"The drive back to Summerton was terrible, ninety minutes in a standard transmission truck, and one of the first things I did when I got home was to contact my primary care doctor—Dr. Mitchell Brodey. Rita telephoned him."

Brodey recalls, "I had taken care of Roy for about seven years, and he'd always been in good health. Because it was unusual for him to call me, I saw him in the office that same day. When he arrived, he looked sick, but I couldn't find a source for his infection on examination."

When a patient consults a doctor for a fever, the physician takes a history and performs a physical examination to determine what, among the literally hundreds of possibilities, might be causing the fever. In this regard, Brodey had an additional advantage. Besides serving as a primary care doctor to his patients, he also has specialized training in infectious diseases. He served as an infectious diseases consultant to local internists and family practitioners. So he would have asked the standard panel of questions: Was there a new rash? A sore throat? Cough or sputum production? Abdominal pain or diarrhea? Burning on urination? And so on. He also would have asked about recent travel to exotic locales, unusual animal or occupational exposure. Next follows the physical examination—is there a swollen liver, or a new heart murmur, a tender prostate or an inflamed joint or red rash?

The combination of the history and the physical examination, along with the context of a case (for example, the season, the patient's age and occupation), will usually point the doctor in one of two directions: a focal process (an infection of a particular organ, as in pneumonia or a urinary tract infection), or a generalized process (an infection that does not settle in any one part of the body, as with a virus that simply leaves a patient feeling run down and showing a fever).

Because the diagnosis was unclear, and the patient looked ill, Brodey admitted Harvey to the local hospital near Syracuse for further diagnostic testing, and to receive intravenous antibiotics, just in case it turned out to be a serious bacterial infection. The other reason for admission was for some old-fashioned observation—a diagnostically useful luxury that modern health economics has all but done away with. Harvey recalls, "Dr. Brodey is probably one of the best doctors you'll ever meet, and I'm glad he's my doctor. He came in to see me [in the hospital]. I was half out of it, but I remember him saying, 'You feel like you're going to die, don't you?' I said, 'You got it,' and he said, 'Well, you're not.'"

One of the tests Brodey ordered was a blood culture, to check for bacteria in the bloodstream.

Later the same day that he admitted Harvey, Brodey was consulted on another patient—a man with a high fever but no true localizing findings in his history or physical examination. "He had spiking fevers, and a headache. As I listened to the story, I remember thinking: 'This story sounds the same as Mr. Harvey's,'" Dr. Brodey says. The two cases piqued his professional curiosity.

A call from the hospital laboratory sated at least part of that curiosity on Friday, July 7. "Roy Harvey's blood culture was positive for *Salmonella typhi*—the causative agent of typhoid fever! I was shocked," recalls Dr. Brodey. "I had been practicing for ten years at that point, and had never seen a case of typhoid." But even though Brodey had made Harvey's diagnosis, the answer only raised more questions.

For instance: How did a man in upstate New York in this day and age get typhoid fever?

Among the more than two thousand types of salmonella bacteria, *Salmonella typhi* is unique; it is the undisputed king of salmonella. The lesser species of salmonella have infiltrated a large portion of our food chain, including chickens and their eggs, pigs, cattle, turtles, snakes, and many others, but *S. typhi* has adapted to only one host—humans. This means that *S. typhi*, a rod-shaped bacterium, does not exist in other animals, as do the lesser salmonella. The bacillus was first observed by Karl Joseph Eberth in 1880, and scientists learned to grown it in artificial culture medium in 1894. Early vaccines were developed shortly thereafter, but these did little to reduce the effects of typhoid fever.

The disease's name derives from the Greek word *typhus*, meaning cloudy, which refers to the stupor patients exhibit from the fevers. Patients infected with typhoid typically suffer blistering fevers, pounding headaches, and sometimes a hacking cough, abdominal pains, constipation or diarrhea, and often a distinctive rash, somewhat poetically named rose spots. But there is nothing at all poetic about typhoid fever.

Over the centuries, the disease has claimed countless lives. During the Civil War, the Confederate armies lost approximately 200,000 soldiers all together—roughly split 25 percent from battle-related casualties and 75 percent from disease, much of which was typhoid fever. In the first edition of a classic medical textbook, *Principles and Practice of Medicine* (1892), Sir William Osler devoted a large section of its 1,050 pages to typhoid—second in length only to the chapter on tuberculosis. The typhoid section detailed his experience with approximately fifteen hundred cases that he personally saw at the Johns Hopkins Hospital. In 1900, typhoid was the most common cause of admission to Boston City Hospital, and the fourth most common cause of death (after tuberculosis, pneumonia, and cancer).

In the seventh edition of the text (1909), Osler wrote: "Typhoid fever has been one of the great scourges of the armies, and kills and maims more than powder or shot. The story of the recent wars forms a sad chapter in human inefficiency. In the Spanish-American War, . . . one fifth of the soldiers in the national encampments had typhoid fever." Typhoid killed 1,580 American troops in that campaign; the enemy killed 243.

Unfortunately typhoid is a problem not just of wartime, nor is it purely of historical interest. The disease is still common in the third world, and cases occur from time to time in industrialized countries too. Of the five hundred or so cases in the United States each year, roughly two-thirds are "imported" by travelers to foreign countries, most commonly in Central America and the Indian subcontinent. Although typhoid is now treatable with antibiotics, 5–10 percent of patients suffer intestinal bleeding, and 1 percent develop the serious complication of bowel perforation. Despite modern medical care and powerful antibiotics, typhoid still carries a 1 percent mortality rate.

Control of typhoid fever, however, as for so many infectious diseases, represents a triumph not of antibiotics but of modern sanitation and public health strategies. After the experience in the Spanish-American War, Dr. Walter Reed drafted a report on typhoid fever in which he concluded: "Indeed, the history of this disease justify us in stating that whenever men congregate and live without adequate provision for disposing of their excrement, there and then typhoid fever will appear." The widespread sanitary practices that were instituted, partly as a result of Reed's report, led to a marked reduction in the importance of typhoid fever as a serious health threat to soldiers in World War I and subsequent wars.

Typhoid fever is a classic food- and water-borne disease, spread by what doctors refer to as the "fecal-oral" route. This somewhat euphemistic expression cannot hide the simple fact that new cases of typhoid fever occur as a result of the organism spreading from the rear end of the intestinal tract of one human being to the front end of another, however circuitously. Epidemics have been linked to sewage, but also to milk, ice cream, meats, canned foods, salads, and even shellfish. The typhoid bacillus will grow temporarily in all of these environments, but the bacteria's only natural reservoir is in people.

Consequently, every typhoid epidemic can be traced ultimately to a human being—either someone suffering from the disease, or an asymptomatic carrier of the bacillus.

One notorious and illustrative example of this principle was an outbreak in Aberdeen, Scotland, in 1964. On Tuesday evening, May 19, 1964, two students with gastrointestinal complaints were transferred from the Aberdeen Royal Infirmary to the city hospital with a clinical suspicion of typhoid fever. A woman had been admitted to the same hospital three days earlier with similar symptoms. The day the two students were transferred, that woman's husband, her two children, and another unrelated boy were also admitted with similar symptoms. The next day, May 20, the first cultures began to return positive for *S. typhi*, and over the following days dozens more patients arrived with the same problem. After taking a history from each of them, the Aberdeen public health physicians found that eleven of the first twelve patients had eaten canned corned beef that had been purchased at a modern supermarket in the city's west end.

Ultimately, 515 patients were afflicted in this epidemic, and 487 were hospitalized, making it one of the largest and certainly one of the most notorious typhoid outbreaks in the twentieth century. Although treated patients often felt improved after days, many were hospitalized for weeks and some for as long as three months in an effort to prevent secondary spread to others. Frequent press conferences were held; the amount of hysteria this outbreak generated was enormous. Aberdeen lost millions of pounds in revenue due to the publicity. Even Queen Elizabeth paid a formal visit on June 28, partly to show her subjects that being in Aberdeen was safe.

Health inspectors traced the path of the canned corned beef, certain that the ultimate source of infection had to have started with a human being. Knowing the incubation period of typhoid fever, the inspectors knew that the contaminated can must have been opened on May 6 or 7. Canned products are heated to temperatures that sterilize their contents, but after this heating process the cans need to be cooled down. The researchers found that, although we think of cans as completely impermeable, in fact they are not. The rapid swings of temperature lead to pressure changes that can create microscopic leaks in their seams. Initially, when the hot cans are placed in cool water, there is a pressure gradient pushing outward from the cans, but as the contents cool, this gradient can reverse, drawing water into the can. If the cooling water is pure, there is no problem; however, if it is not, impurities can enter the can.

The Aberdeen corned beef had been imported from Argentina. The canning plant was located on the Parana River, just downstream from the city of Rosario, with a population of more than 600,000 people. The city's sewage was discharged into the river, and the nearest sewage discharge pipe was about half a mile upstream from the factory. Investigators estimated that every day 66 tons of excrement and 250,000 gallons of urine passed by the plant. The fast-flowing Parana River at Rosario is about 50 feet deep and 1,300 yards wide, so the sewage was considerably diluted. But the incidence of typhoid in Argentina in the 1960s was approximately 500 cases per million inhabitants (in Britain at the same time, it was 2). A single typhoid carrier can excrete millions of bacteria per day. So it is very possible that typhoid bacilli, which are known to survive in river water, were present as the water flowed past the factory. And here, the Rosario canning plant draws its water to cool the cans after they are heat sterilized.

Incredibly, in 1955, another outbreak of typhoid in Great Britain, at Pickering, was linked to tongue meat that had been canned at the very same plant in Rosario. As a direct result of that epidemic, the Argentine plant began to chlorinate the cooling water. In 1962, however, there had been a breakdown in the chlorination process that, for various economic and logistical reasons, had never been fixed. So despite the history of the Pickering outbreak, at the time of the Aberdeen epidemic, the cooling water from the river was untreated and almost certainly contained *S. typhi*.

But if *S. typhi* was getting into the cans, one would expect them to also contain other bacteria that are far more plentiful, especially *Escherichia coli*. It is for this reason that another quality control is implemented in the canning process. After the cans are cooled and washed, they are observed for fifteen days. The purpose of this step is to watch for "blown cans." Any *E. coli* that has entered the cans will rapidly multiply. This produces gas that pushes out the walls of the cans, making them appear "blown" from the inside. Also, once a can like this is opened, it is usually obvious that the meat has gone bad, so the consumer will smell and see that the food is contaminated, and not eat it.

This notion was dispelled following the Aberdeen epidemic of 1964, however, when on June 1, some normal-appearing cans of corned beef from Argentina were cultured. Although the meat appeared wholesome and the cans were not blown, both *E. coli* and *S. typhi* were found in the meat. The other interesting finding was that only a portion of the meat grew the bacteria, and other samples from the same can were sterile, so it was possible that a small amount of contamination had occurred but the conditions in the can were not conducive to further growth (which would presumably explain why the cans were not blown). Could this have caused the illnesses in Aberdeen?

An investigation later revealed that, once the original six-pound can of corned beef had been opened at the supermarket, some of the contents were placed in the cold-meats counter, and some in a south-facing display window in the store. Meteorological records showed that it was warm in Aberdeen for the days of May 7–9, and the meat in the south-facing window provided ideal conditions for *S. typhi* to multiply. And *S. typhi* loves to multiply; several bacteria can grow into several million in a matter of hours. The connection between a human source from Rosario, Argentina, and the contaminated food source in Aberdeen, Scotland, had been established.

Dr. Brodey's first thought was the lab result on Roy Harvey's blood had to be a mistake. After all, he had been a practicing infectious diseases specialist for a decade and had never encountered a case of typhoid fever. But then the blood culture from the second patient, whose story sounded so much like Harvey's, turned positive for *S. typhi* as well. "At that point," recalls Dr. Brodey, "I knew something was going on. I re-interviewed both men at length; neither had been out of the country. These second interviews revealed one important connection, however. Both men were firefighters, and both had been to the convention in the Catskills." Since his experience with typhoid had just rocketed from zero in ten years to two cases in a day, Brodey feared this might be the tip of an iceberg.

He promptly notified the New York State Health Department in Albany.

"Like every outbreak," remembers Stan Kondracki somewhat facetiously, "it was reported on a Friday night." In 1989, Kondracki was the co-coordinator of the New York state regional epidemiology program. "We had the county people ship the diagnostic specimens from the two patients to the state lab in Albany for confirmation of typhoid. Over the weekend, we got that confirmation and the investigation started Monday morning. It was an epidemiologist's delight, but required lots of work. The Fire Chiefs' Association sent us a computer printout of the names and phone numbers of all the conventioneers. The hotels gave us lists of the other guests. There were senior citizens groups from Ohio, Connecticut, and Pennsylvania, as well as individual guests. We drafted staff from the AIDS and sexually transmitted diseases sections to help with all of the interviews and telephone calls."

In fact, the team included a large number of individuals not only from the New York State Department of Health's Bureau of Communicable Diseases but also from its sanitation, food protection, and laboratory groups. Other important help was supplied by various district and local public health agencies, as well as the Sullivan County Public Health nursing services. Last, an epidemiology intelligence officer from the CDC in Atlanta rounded out the team. There was plenty of work for everyone. Says Kondracki, "We needed to establish the usual things: time, place, and person."

And they needed to establish these parameters quickly. The first round of phone calls showed that the scope of the problem was growing rapidly, with cases popping up throughout the state. Kondracki and his colleagues' first steps were to design and distribute surveys to a large group of people. There were almost ten thousand firefighters who had stayed at six different hotels in the area, in addition to all of the other guests. Performing the survey and analyzing the data was no small task. The surveys quickly yielded an important piece of information. All of the typhoid patients had stayed in a single hotel (which I'll call Grovers). "The hotel management was extremely cooperative," recalls Kondracki. "We obtained a guest list for the period just prior to and immediately following the June 11–14 convention time."

Another salvo of telephone calls helped to narrow down the time frame. Only guests staying at Grovers during the convention developed typhoid, but not all of them. Kondracki had the time and place, but he still needed to pin down the exact persons. Why did some guests staying at Grovers between June 11 and 14 fall ill while others did not? To answer that question, the epidemiologists examined the two most likely potential sources—the water and the food. Grovers used the municipal water supply, which was quickly tested and ruled out as a source. The plumbing was also checked to make sure there was no cross-contamination between a sewer pipe and a clean water source. This also proved to be a dead end.

The investigators had already surveyed the hotel guests about which meals they had taken at the hotel and which foods they had eaten at those meals. This was a formidable job: the hotel had 450 rooms with a capacity of 800 guests, as well as approximately 250 employees, half of whom work in food service. After analyzing the surveys, the investigators pinned down the particular meal that had caused the illness with surgical precision.

All of the people who developed typhoid had eaten breakfast at Grovers on the morning of Tuesday, June 13.

But there were still critical questions that needed answering. Roy Harvey had eaten breakfast at Grovers that morning, but so had Rita Harvey, and she was still perfectly well. After an initial rally, Roy's condition deteriorated. By his third day in the hospital, his fever broke, and he began to feel better. He was even hoping to be discharged the following Monday, July 10. But over the weekend, he developed one of the feared complications of typhoid—intestinal bleeding. The inflammation had burrowed into the richly vascular lymphoid tissue in his small intestine. When the infection eroded deep enough into these blood vessels, he began to bleed. "When I looked in the toilet bowl, it was filled with bright red blood," he remembers. "I called Heather, the nurse, and she helped me back to bed. I had lost about half my blood and needed a transfusion. I remember there were informed consent forms to sign.

"I didn't want to get the blood, but she said it was either that or possibly bleed to death. When she put it that way, the choice was easy. I got four pints," said Harvey.

The New York epidemiologists had their goal clearly in mind—to find the source and to prevent more cases. To accomplish this, the investigators still had two important tasks to complete. The first was to identify the specific item at breakfast that had been contaminated. The second was to find out just how the typhoid bacillus got there.

Grovers' food service was a large operation. There was a main kitchen and a coffee shop that, combined, served three thousand meals per day, with more than eighty menu items. The answer to the first question came rapidly; the food surveys distributed to the guests answered it unequivocally. But the food that the questionnaires implicated seemed very unlikely: orange juice. This was a surprise because the natural acidity of orange juice makes it a very unlikely vehicle to support the growth of S. typhi.

The second job, to determine precisely how the typhoid got into the juice, remained elusive. Questionnaires would not solve this dilemma; that would require some old-fashioned shoe-leather detective work.

Nearly all the hotel employees had cultures taken to test for typhoid. One worker, who was of interest to the investigation, had left Grovers shortly after the convention, on June 21. Of the remaining 250 workers, only one, a man I'll call George Watkins, tested positive for S. typhi. Watkins was a dishwasher, but he occasionally helped prepare the orange juice, and he always drank several glasses each morning. Watkins' stool cultures grew the bacterium only for about a week after the outbreak, and then they turned negative in follow-up tests, and remained that way. The transient positive result suggested that he may have been a victim of the outbreak, rather than its source. If he had been a carrier, he would most likely have remained culture positive, and his blood test for antibodies (which was negative) would most likely have been positive too. The worker who had left the employ of Grovers was a breakfast cook who had been in charge of making the orange juice. He did so by emptying twenty-four thirty-two-ounce cans of juice concentrate into a fifty-five-gallon plastic drum, similar to a large trash can. He would then add twenty-four gallons of water and stir the mixture with a wire whisk.

Every typhoid outbreak begins with a human excreting the typhoid bacillus through the stool (or, rarely, in the urine). The infected stool might come from a person who is sick with or recovering from an acute infection with typhoid fever, or, more commonly, from a carrier of the typhoid bacteria. The carrier state is an interesting balance that is struck between pathogen (in this case, *S. typhi*) and host (in this case, someone who has been naturally infected with the typhoid bacillus). Roughly 3 percent of typhoid patients become carriers.

The pioneering Prussian physician and microbiologist Robert Koch first suggested the concept of a typhoid carrier. He presented his hypothesis in a talk in Berlin on November 28, 1902, after observing that a small percentage of patients recovering from typhoid continued to shed the bacilli for months after recovery. The concept of a carrier was a novel, still unproved theory. Typhoid carriers persistently shed typhoid bacteria in their stools, even though they are not ill. If sewage contaminated with typhoid makes its way into drinking water, or if a carrier prepares food without thoroughly washing his hands after going to the bathroom, the bacillus can spread like wildfire.

In the Aberdeen epidemic, some patients became sick, not from eating the contaminated corned beef, but from eating other meats that had been cut with the same knife!

Without doubt the most famous typhoid carrier in history is "Typhoid Mary," born Mary Mallon in Cookstown, County Tyrone, Ireland, on September 23, 1869. At the age of fourteen, the tall, stocky blonde moved to New York City, where she began working as a cook. Her employment record was abysmal; she hopped from job to job.

Toward the end of August 1906, the daughter of a wealthy New York banker, Charles Henry Warren, developed typhoid fever. The family summered in fashionable Oyster Bay, Long Island, where they rented a large property. When five other members of the household quickly fell ill with typhoid too, local health officials investigated. They found no contaminated food, water, or milk, so, having come up empty-handed, they closed the investigation.

The owner of the house, concerned that he would be unable to rent the place the next summer, hired Dr. George Soper, a sanitary engineer with the New York City Health Department and a recognized typhoid expert, to investigate further. Soper followed standard procedures, first verifying the results of the previous investigation. There being no demonstrable source of the bacteria in any food or drink at the house, or in the plumbing (both indoor and outdoor), Soper considered the possibility of a typhoid carrier. He hoped to confirm Koch's theory. He learned that the Warren family had recently hired a cook, one Mary Mallon, and he wanted to find her.

One senses Soper's excitement from his own description of that quest.

First I went to the employment agency where I was given the missing cook's former places of employment and the different people who had furnished her with references. Working from agency to agency I came in possession of little fragments of her history for ten years. What do you suppose I found out? That in every household in which she had worked in the last ten years, there had been an outbreak of typhoid fever. Mind you, there wasn't a single exception.

The question that confronted me now was: "Where is she?" Following her trail backward to cases in 1904, I found she had worked at the home of Henry Gilsey at Sands Point, Long Island, where four of seven servants suddenly got the disease. Going back still further, I found that five weeks after Mary had gone to cook at the home of J. Coleman Drayton at Dark Harbor, Maine, in 1902, seven out of nine persons in the house contracted typhoid, and so did a trained nurse and a woman who came to the house to work by the day. There had been an outbreak of the disease in New York in 1901, and I had reason to believe that Mary was behind this. In 1904, Tuxedo Park, the fashionable summer resort, was stricken, . . . and [I] discovered she had cooked there in that time.

Finally Soper got the break he needed. Just days after leaving the employ of the Warrens in Oyster Bay, Mary had taken a job on September 21, 1906, in Tuxedo, New York. Typhoid soon followed, but Mary left the household before Soper could find her. Then, in March 1907, Soper was hired to investigate a typhoid outbreak in a fashionable New York brownstone, the home of Walter Bowen at 688 Park Avenue. Soper finally found Mary Mallon and confronted her. According to his account, "I had my first talk with Mary in the kitchen of this house. . . . I was as diplomatic as possible, but I had to say I suspected her of making people sick and that I wanted specimens of her urine, feces, and blood. It did not take Mary long to react to this suggestion. She seized a carving fork and advanced in my direction. I passed rapidly down the hall, through the tall iron gate . . . and so to the sidewalk. I felt rather lucky to escape."

Soper then tracked Mary down to a rooming house and returned with a colleague, but, despite "as much tact and judgment as we possessed," they could not persuade her to submit to an examination. The New York health commissioner interceded, and a group including a female physician, Dr. Josephine Baker, accompanied by the police, went to arrest Mary. Mallon greeted them once again sporting a "long kitchen fork in her hand like a rapier," wrote Dr. Baker. "As she lunged at me with the fork, I stepped back, recoiled on the policemen, and so confused matters that by the time we had got through the door, Mary had disappeared." She hid in a closet, but a scrap of her blue calico dress, caught in the closet door, drew their attention.

According to Dr. Baker, a thin, bespectacled woman, "She came out fighting and swearing, both of which she could do with appalling efficiency and vigor. . . . She knew that she had never had typhoid fever; she was maniacal in her integrity. There was nothing to do but to take her with us. They lifted her into the ambulance and I literally sat on her all the way to the hospital; it was like being in a cage with an angry lion."

Mallon was placed in an isolation ward of the Willard Parker Hospital, a contagious disease unit in New York. From Mary's perspective, the notion that she could be spreading the disease was nonsense. She had never been sick with typhoid; she must have had a very mild case that mimicked some other minor illness back when she lived in Ireland. Nevertheless, her initial cultures, as well as those taken over the ensuing eight months, all grew out typhoid bacilli. She is generally believed to be the first documented case of an asymptomatic typhoid carrier in the United States. The city health department offered her surgical removal of the gallbladder, on the theory that the typhoid bacilli settled there in carriers. Mary, not ignorant of the risks of that surgical procedure in 1907, refused the operation.

Because health authorities were not convinced that Mary Mallon would obey their directive that she not work as a food handler or cook, she was confined in quarantine at Riverside Hospital, a small, isolated institution on North Brother Island, a thirteen-acre patch of earth in the East River (near the present site of La Guardia Airport). A very public legal battle ensued, highlighting the classic conflict between personal liberty and the public good. Lawyers tried to free her, but the courts upheld the state's legal right to hold her involuntarily, arguing that she represented an "imminent peril." The city officials cited two sections of the Greater New York Charter that read:

> *The board of health shall use all reasonable means for ascertaining the existence and cause of disease or peril to life or health, and for averting the same, throughout the city. [Section 1169]*
>
> *Said board may remove or cause to be removed to a proper place to be by it designated, any person sick with any contagious, pestilential or infectious disease; shall have exclusive charge and control of the hospital for the treatment of such cases. [Section 1170]*

In the press coverage following the legal case, the media dubbed Mallon "Typhoid Mary." Typhoid was a common cause of death during the early years of the twentieth century; the public had little patience with someone who knowingly spread the disease to others. It would be akin to someone nowadays knowingly exposing people to HIV or a resistant strain of tuberculosis.

On February 19, 1910, Mary was released after promising to change jobs and be monitored by the health authorities. She did neither, and more small outbreaks were attributed to her. Again, Soper apprehended her (in 1915), and again she was held involuntarily. She remained quarantined at Riverside Hospital for the rest of her life. She died of a stroke in 1938, having spent half her life in confinement.

Mary Mallon was personally responsible for at least 53 cases of typhoid fever and three deaths. At the time of her death, there were 349 other typhoid carriers known in New York City, but she was the only one who was confined; the others simply changed their habits and submitted to regular monitoring by the health authorities. Although other carriers, such as "Mr. N," a cow milker from Folkestone, England, are responsible for spreading the disease more widely (to approximately two hundred people in his case), Mary Mallon is by far the most notorious.

In the Catskill outbreak among the firefighters, both the water supply and the hotel plumbing system had been tested and exonerated as the source of the bacteria. That left the missing breakfast cook, who, as it turned out, proved even more difficult to locate than Typhoid Mary.

Says Kondracki, "Gone are the days where college students work the Catskills. The breakfast cook who left was from Central America, where typhoid is endemic and typhoid carriers are more common. We suspect, but could never prove, that he was the source. He left Grovers before the outbreak hit the news. We tried to track him down in several ways. A Spanish-speaking public health nurse even staked out his last known New York address, but he never showed up there. We also corresponded with Social Security and the welfare folks, but we never found him."

Despite the failure to locate the cook, Kondracki is still pretty sure he knows precisely how the bacteria got into the orange juice. "People respond to interviews differently," he recalls. "The first time I interviewed Watkins [the infected dishwasher], he was in the kitchen with his boss present. He was very closed mouthed. Later, I spoke with him without his boss [being present]. I took him for a stroll outside the building, and we sat at a picnic table on the side lawn and just shot the breeze a bit. When it was clear to him that I wasn't a police-type person, he opened up. He told me that they stirred the orange juice with a two-foot-long metal whisk. I remember him saying 'it was the one with the string on it,' although I wasn't sure what he meant at the time.

"When I returned to the kitchen, there were three metal whisks hanging from the wall. One of them had a piece of string that attached the handle to the whisk. I confiscated it although I knew I'd never culture anything out since it had been though the dishwasher at 180 degrees. As I was driving out of town, I bumped into Watkins on a street corner, quite by accident. I pulled over, opened the trunk and asked him if the whisk with the string [that I had confiscated] was the one he and the missing cook had used. It was.

"I asked him why the string was there. He told me it was to keep the whisk attached to the handle. It had kept falling off [without the string]," Kondracki says, his voice now filling with excitement. "You see the point. When it fell into the orange juice, he would have to reach his arm into the plastic bin to retrieve the thing. That established in my mind the connection. His workstation was right outside the employee's bathroom, which was not equipped with soap and water or paper towels. I had a plausible biological explanation."

To address the problem that the juice was an unusual vehicle, the state investigators performed lab experiments using the same strain of ty-phoid found in the epidemic, along with the orange juice, which has a very acidic pH of 3.8. They found that, although the bacteria would die in less than two hours in the orange juice concentrate, they could live for more than six hours in the reconstituted (and more diluted) juice. The report goes on to state, "Theoretical calculations of the infective dose showed that 30–50 gallons of orange juice could have been contami-nated with 50 mg [a miniscule amount] of fecal material, and still have achieved sufficient numbers of organisms in a glass of orange juice to cause illness."

Ultimately, forty-five confirmed cases were identified, making the Catskill outbreak the largest domestic typhoid epidemic in nearly a decade. Besides the confirmed cases, twenty-four others were strongly suspected to be involved but were never proved with certainty. Includ-ing both groups, the attack rate was 11 percent of hotel guests at Grovers.

Twenty-one patients were sick enough to require hospitalization. Four developed complications: two cases of gastrointestinal bleeding and two of bowel perforation, which requires surgery. Fortunately no-body died in this epidemic.

Roy Harvey, after four blood transfusions and a ten-day hospitaliza-tion, survived, although he remained out of work for four weeks. As for Rita, who never got sick, her husband explains, "She's just not a juice drinker."

~~~~~~~~~~~~~~~~~~~~~~~~

It began on June 15, 1988, as one of the most routine cases in a pediatrician's practice. After all, there are few problems more common than a toddler with diarrhea.

At first, fourteen-month-old Katie Wolz of Cape Girardeau, Missouri, developed her diarrhea without any other symptoms, not even a fever—just diarrhea. Her mother, Kathleen Wolz, an energetic thirty-year-old lawyer, reacted the same way most moms would. "I thought it was one of those viruses that kids are always getting," she recalls. "She didn't look sick, so I put her on liquids and figured it would pass." But a few days later, it hadn't passed. Little Katie still had diarrhea and now had begun spiking fevers to 102 degrees. "It was the middle of the summer and really hot. I was afraid she'd get dehydrated, so I took her to the pediatrician," her mom remembers.

So on July 20, Dr. Jesse R. Ramsey, a pediatrician in Cape Girardeau, examined Katie. He found her to be in good health and without any signs of serious dehydration. He concluded that the most likely diagnosis was a simple gastroenteritis.

Bacteria and other microorganisms have a limited number of methods for entering the human body. One route is through the skin after it is abraded or cut, which provides an opening for the bacteria that normally lurk on the outside of the skin. The result is often a skin infection called cellulitis. Other times, a microorganism can gain access to the bloodstream through intact skin that is penetrated by the bite of a mosquito or a tick. Malaria and Lyme disease are examples of this mechanism. Another point of entrance is the respiratory system; numerous viruses and bacteria attack by this mode, hitching a ride on the very air we breathe. Tuberculosis and influenza are two bugs that attack in this manner, but there are countless others. Occasionally, microorganisms can get inside humans by penetrating mucous membranes like the eyes, throat, or genital tract. Conjunctivitis, strep tonsillitis, and syphilis are examples of attack through these routes.

And then, of course, there is the gastrointestinal tract. Every morsel of food and every sip of a drink that we place into our mouths has the potential of carrying pathogenic hitchhikers. Most of those are inactivated by the acidity in the stomach. Others cannot withstand the assault of various digestive enzymes in the stomach and intestines. And still others are hunted down and destroyed by special immunoglobulins that are found in the gut. But in spite of this multilayered protective strategy, some pathogens overwhelm the host defense mechanisms, and when they do, they often produce the common syndrome of gastroenteritis.

Gastroenteritis is a generic term that encompasses a host of different afflictions of the gastrointestinal tract; the condition is one of humanity's most common ailments. It is usually heralded by nausea, vomiting, and fever, which is soon followed by abdominal cramping and diarrhea. Gastroenteritis can be caused by a wide variety of pathogens—bacteria, viruses, and parasites as well as toxins and poisons. The majority of patients improve rapidly and without antibiotics. Generally, after several days of bed rest, lots of clear liquids, and avoiding dairy products, the body successfully combats the invading microorganism or toxin and the tide of the battle tilts toward a favorable outcome for the patient.

On the other hand, when the organism is a particularly vicious one, say cholera or typhoid, and when hydration cannot be accomplished, the resulting complications of fluid loss can be disastrous and in some cases fatal. In the third world in 1980, 4.6 million children died from dehydration that resulted from diarrhea. This mind-boggling number was reduced to 3.1 million in 1990, in large part due to the use of oral rehydration therapy that diminished the need for intravenous hydration, a prohibitively expensive and logistically difficult treatment in much of the underdeveloped world. The underlying diseases can sometimes be controlled by the body's defense mechanisms, but if the person cannot keep up with hydration, even a "self-limiting" disease can be fatal.

Although this progress has been impressive, diarrhea remains one of the most common causes of child mortality in the world. Even in the United States, the CDC estimates that food-borne diseases cause approximately 76 million illnesses, 325,000 hospitalizations, and 5,000 deaths each year. The deaths are usually in patients who have problems with their immune systems, are very old, or are very young.

But Katie Wolz was not in the third world; this was Cape Girardeau, Missouri, in the heartland of America. And she had a perfectly normal immune system. Katie didn't appear critically ill from the infection, and she was keeping down the necessary fluids, so Dr. Ramsey quite properly decided to hold off on antibiotics, and reassured Mrs. Wolz that she was already taking all the right steps. At the same time, however, he was sufficiently concerned by the persistence of fever and diarrhea; Katie had been ill for several days, enough time that Dr. Ramsey would have expected to see some improvement in many routine cases. There are approximately two hundred different diseases that can be spread through the gastrointestinal system, and knowing the specific cause can help identify the correct treatment. So Dr. Ramsey ordered a stool sample to be analyzed by the lab for the presence of various microorganisms—a perfectly routine test.

Two days later, he received a call back from the lab with a result that was anything but routine. There was good news and bad news.

The good news was that the specimen was negative for the usual pathogens. Rotavirus is an extremely common viral pathogen causing acute gastroenteritis in children younger than five. It gives rise to about three million cases of diarrhea each year in the United States and results in about fifty-five thousand hospitalizations. But rotavirus is usually a winter disease, and it is very contagious. This was summer, and none of Katie's friends were ill.

The rotavirus test was negative. The culture was also negative for the usual bacterial pathogens that the laboratory normally tests for—salmonella, campylobacter, and shigella. So much for the good news.

The bad news, or to put the most optimistic spin on it, the surprising news, was that "an unusual" bacteria was growing. "In fact, it was one I had never heard of before," recalls Ramsey, "*Plesiomonas shigelloides.* I quickly looked it up and learned that the bacterium was extremely rare in the United States, but far more common in the tropics. My initial reaction was, 'I don't believe it; this has got to be a mistake,'" says Dr.

Ramsey. "But I couldn't be sure, so I asked the lab to forward the sample to the state lab in Jefferson City for confirmation." Then he telephoned Mrs. Wolz.

"It was one of those 'Don't be alarmed, but' phone calls that you really love to get from your doctor," she remembers. "He told me that Katie's culture was growing a rare bacteria and that he had notified the state lab. What frightened me was that nobody seemed sure what to do. But Katie, although she still was having some diarrhea, was much better and had no fever. I was reassured by that. Dr. Ramsey also said that he was going to get the health department involved."

Sue Tippen is a communicable diseases coordinator for the Missouri Department of Health, in the southeastern district, headquartered in Poplar Bluff. Along with all the mundane scraps of paper that find their way to her desk each day was the results of Katie Wolz's stool culture. That report stood out from all the others on that summer day because, like most health care professionals, she too had never heard of *Plesiomonas shigelloides*. So Tippen did a little research on the subject. Even in the library, she wasn't able to find out very much, but one thing seemed clear: the bacteria with the long name had no business showing up in her jurisdiction.

Tucked away on the banks of the Mississippi River, about 120 miles south of St. Louis, Cape Girardeau is a college town of about 40,000 inhabitants, many of whom are associated with Southeastern Missouri State University. Though it's not an active port, an occasional riverboat loaded with tourists ties up at its docks. And although the town might serve as a perfect setting for a Mark Twain story, Cape Girardeau is not particularly exotic, and certainly anything but tropical.

That's what baffled Sue Tippen as she examined the report in front of her. As she put it, "I don't expect subtropical diseases to be reported in southeastern Missouri."

Plesiomonas shigelloides, which, to preserve the reader's sanity, I'll simply refer to as PS, is an unusual bacterium in this country. A relative newcomer to the stage of microorganisms, at least in terms of when humans catalogued it, it was first described in 1947. It was thought to be a close cousin to the more notorious cholera bacillus. Cholera is caused by the bacterium *Vibrio cholera*, which was first discovered back in 1883 by the renowned bacteriologist Robert Koch. Known for its large epidemics (an outbreak in London in 1849 killed 14,137 people, and another in 1854 killed more than 5 percent of Chicago's population), cholera is not only of historical interest. The disease is still endemic in many parts of the world. Beginning in 1991, an outbreak that lasted several years affected more than a million persons and killed nearly ten thousand. Even in the United States, sporadic cases and small clusters of cholera still occur, generally in people in the Gulf states who have been eating raw shellfish.

As recently as 1998, the Colorado Department of Public Health and Environment was notified of a case of cholera in a seventy-three-year-old woman who had never traveled out of state. On September 19, the patient and eleven family members ate blue crabs that had been harvested along the Gulf Coast, precooked, and commercially distributed by a Louisiana company. Two days after the meal, the patient developed profuse watery diarrhea and nausea, and was hospitalized. Her stool culture was positive for *Vibrio cholera.*

PS, like its more famous vibrio relative, very rarely causes disease in the United States. Initially it was lumped with the vibrios, but over time doctors learned that PS was biochemically distinct from the true vibrios, even though there are similarities between the two bacteria.

One survey conducted by the CDC in Atlanta detected only thirty-one cases of PS in a one-year period in the entire United States. Some investigators feel that it is more common than that but some cases may go undiagnosed, which certainly might have happened with Katie Wolz had Dr. Ramsey not ordered the culture in the first place. The CDC group found that PS infections in the country are associated with eating undercooked shellfish or recent travel to areas with warmer climates, especially Mexico and the Caribbean.

A Canadian study arrived at similar conclusions. Like their American counterparts, these researchers found that many of their patients had traveled to tropical locales. A significant minority had never left British Columbia, however; most of those patients had eaten raw shellfish, mostly oysters. This link with eating undercooked shellfish, especially oysters, is also seen in patients with domestically acquired cholera. Most of the patients in both of these studies suffered from diarrhea, severe abdominal cramping, and fever. Some had gastrointestinal bleeding as well. In both studies, the largest that exist, nearly all of the patients with PS had either traveled abroad or eaten undercooked shellfish.

A group of Japanese investigators looked for PS in many different environments in and around Tokyo. Not only did they find PS in an occasional patient with gastroenteritis, but they were also able to culture the organism from 4 percent of dogs and 10 percent of cats. They also found the bug in 10 to 12 percent of samples of river water and sludge from riverbanks in the Tokyo area. This link with animals extends beyond dogs and cats. The bacterium has been found in freshwater fish, poultry, cows, pigs, even snakes.

And snakes from Japan are not the only ones to harbor the bacterium. One such serpentine example occurred in the case of an American man, a twenty-one-year-old employee in the animal research division at the National Zoo in Washington who had been caring for a boa constrictor that was ill with mouth-rot disease. The snake died, and the employee helped perform the autopsy. During the procedure, he wore a gown and gloves. About twenty hours later, on July 15, 1976, he developed nausea, vomiting, chills, profuse watery diarrhea, severe abdominal cramps, and low-grade fever. He was sick enough to go the emergency room at Georgetown University Hospital. He had a temperature of 100.4 degrees Fahrenheit and a fast pulse and showed signs of dehydration. The treating doctors sent off a stool culture.

When the man was still sick five days later, he returned to the hospital. The stool culture that had been taken on the first visit was now growing PS. Cultures from the snake obtained both before its death and at autopsy were also positive for organisms suggestive of PS. The man was treated with antibiotics for a week and recovered. In fact, most healthy adults with PS infections experience relatively mild symptoms that resolve without treatment. Others, however, like the zoo employee, need antibiotics and some are sufficiently ill to require hospitalization.

Most PS infections in humans involve the gastrointestinal tract, but the bacteria have also caused infections of the skin, joints, gallbladder, and bloodstream. On rare occasions, it can cause meningitis. In 1983, a three-day-old infant was diagnosed with meningitis. The pregnancy and delivery had gone without a hitch, but on day two of its life the child rapidly became blue and had diffuse contractures of his tiny muscles. He was given antibiotics and transferred to a pediatric ICU early the next day. On admission to the ICU, he had a cardiac arrest, but was resuscitated. A spinal tap revealed meningitis and PS was cultured from the spinal fluid and the bloodstream. At age four and a half days, he died. The precise source of the PS was never found. Although this case is exceptionally rare, it does show that PS can be a very dangerous bug.

Because PS infection is not a reportable disease in Missouri (or in most other states either), Tippen was not officially required to pursue the matter any further. "But it piqued my interest," she explained, "so I decided to investigate anyway. I phoned Mrs. Wolz to get some background information."

"Sue Tippen called me at work one day," recalls Kathy Wolz. "She asked me if we had been out of the country and I laughed. With my schedule, we hardly go anywhere. Then we talked about other potential sources of Katie's infection. We had visited a local swimming spot, Kentucky Lake, on July Fourth weekend, but the weather hadn't been good, and Katie had barely been in the water, just splashed around some. We swam at another private lake in the next county around the same time, but I didn't think Katie had drank any of the water or got any in her mouth, although I couldn't be completely sure."

After the first salvo of questions failed to provide much in the way of clues, Tippen then followed with a whole array of others. In her mind, she was trying to track down the source of the odd bacteria. Was it in the water? In the environment? The food? She pursued the investigation in several directions. She learned that the child drank only municipal water, and since no other cases had been reported in the area, that seemed an extremely unlikely source. She learned that the family's only pet was a cocker spaniel named Maverick, and Maverick was perfectly healthy. Then they discussed food. Of course it came as no surprise that neither oysters nor other undercooked shellfish (or any other suspicious food) had been on the toddler's menu. When Tippen found out that Katie attended a day care center, which seemed like a definite lead, she decided to investigate the site in person. "The director of the facility was not at all happy," recalls Mrs. Wolz, who made that phone call. But as is usually the case in such situations, the director cooperated fully.

"My records indicate that I visited the day care center on August 12," recalls Tippen, looking through her case file. "I spoke with several of the day care personnel. I found a clean, church-run facility with about a hundred children enrolled. In looking for any possible source of the PS, I did note that some guinea pigs were kept in a room where the older children congregated. But there were no animals in the infant room, where Katie and about ten other youngsters played. Furthermore, none of those other children at the facility were sick with similar illnesses as Katie's."

If the gastroenteritis had developed at the day care center, then it would be expected that there would be more than one case, and Katie was the only child who was ill. But Tippen learned about one other interesting fact on her site visit that day. There was a second connection between Katie and the day care center. One of the employees, a twenty-year-old named Marci Mann, babysat for Katie each Tuesday evening. Normally she would take care of Katie at the Wolz home. But occasionally, for some scheduling reason or another, Marci would bring Katie to her apartment. Tippen casually inquired about any animals at Marci's place and learned that yes, Marci and her husband, Kevin, did keep several pets—a cat, and an aquarium stocked with five piranhas!

"We bought them from a tropical fish store in St. Louis, and we feed them minnows," said Marci.

With this, Tippen felt a pulse of excitement rush through her body. She knew that piranhas were the infamous flesh-eating fish from the Amazon River basin in South America—distinctly tropical. She also knew that other scientists had isolated PS from fish tanks. In one British study done a year before, investigators took samples from one hundred fish tanks in six pet shops in the Cardiff area. A full 100 percent of the aquariums contained some kind of pathological bacteria. Salmonella species were found in only eight of the tanks, but *Aeromonas* species (a bacterium closely related to PS), was found in ninety-eight of the tanks. And PS was found in one.

So the connection with an aquarium and tropical fish was quite possibly the missing link that Sue Tippen had been searching for.

Yet there were problems with the piranha theory from the start. First, the fish were in excellent health, although Tippen knew that this was frequently the case with diseases carried by animals and transmitted to humans. A bigger difficulty was that Marci and her husband kept the aquarium on a high shelf, and it also had a sturdy, tight-fitting cover over it. Toddlers are notorious for their Houdini-like skills, but there simply was no way that Katie could have gotten into the fish tank. Although Tippen felt sure that the piranhas had to be involved, she couldn't see how, and the investigation seemed to come to a dead end.

But not for long.

"A couple of weeks later," said Mrs. Wolz, "on a Tuesday evening when I entered Marci's apartment to pick up Katie, I noticed something curious. Marci had just gotten Katie out of the bathtub. What struck me had nothing to do with Marci or Katie, but Marci's husband. Kevin was feeding the fish. Because the subject of fish had come up in our conversations with Sue Tippen, Marci and I started talking about them. I hadn't even known that they kept fish. I remember saying to her, 'there's no way Katie could get up there.' Then Kevin began to clean the tank, and it was clear he was about to dump some of the water into the tub. The aquarium has a filter, but every so often, they would dump the water into the tub. That was because they live on a second-floor apartment, and the tub was the logical place to dump it. It still didn't ring any bells.

"Then all of a sudden, it just clicked. Marci and I looked at each other and said at the same time, 'the bathtub!' Katie loves to drink water from the tub," Mrs. Wolz explained. "She especially likes to suck on the wet wash cloth; we always joke about it."

They quickly notified Sue Tippen, who, armed with this new fact, sent some sample bottles to Marci, who filled them with water from the fish tank. On August 23, she forwarded the water specimens to the state lab in Jefferson City to be analyzed for PS.

Fish can transmit several diseases to humans, mainly when eaten as food. Sushi is associated with various parasites, especially a tiny round worm that causes abdominal pain and diarrhea, a disorder called anisakiasis. Sometimes the pain is severe, and it has been misdiagnosed as a stomach ulcer or appendicitis. The fish tapeworm can also be transmitted by eating fish; years ago, this was not uncommon in Jewish grandmothers from New York as they tasted their gefilte fish before it was fully prepared. Far rarer is contracting botulism from eating fish. Toxins from fish can lead to scombroid and ciguatera poisoning and paralytic fish poisoning.

Handling fish can also lead to infections. There is a form of skin infection (cellulitis) that is due to a bacterium with another hard-to-pronounce name, *Erysipelothrix*. It's important for doctors to consider this somewhat unusual cause since it responds to different antibiotics than are usually used for cellulitis. Certain vibrio species can also cause a severe cellulitis, including one called *Vibrio vulnificus*. This bug is generally spread via contact on abraded skin. The skin infection that results is associated with huge blisters that can cause the skin to slough off. It is especially severe in immunocompromised patients or those with liver disease, where it can sometimes lead to severe sepsis and death. These vibrio infections are most commonly associated with uncooked or raw shellfish, leading some to suggest that immunocompromised individuals should be very cautious when eating oysters and the like.

But can people get infections from the fish or the water in an aquarium? The answer is a resounding yes, although it does not happen very often. In the United States more than 20 million households have aquariums. Each year, approximately 600 million pet fish are sold in this country. These fish mostly come from Southeast Asia and South America. In spite of these enormous numbers, no major outbreaks of human disease from diseased aquarium fish have ever been reported.

One type of infection that people can get from their aquariums is called aquarium finger, swimming pool granuloma, or fish tuberculosis. The bacteria responsible are *Mycobacterium marinum*, which is closely related to the one that causes human tuberculosis. This infection can be acquired from swimming pools or aquariums, and from handling fish. Because the bacterium is more active at lower temperatures, it usually causes a skin infection characterized by exuberant growth of tissue called a granuloma.

The most frequent sign is a slowly developing nodule on the skin. Because the organism is suited to the temperature of the fish and not humans, it usually affects cooler parts of the body, such as a finger, hand, or arm. Later the nodule can enlarge and ulcerate. Nearby lymph nodes swell. Although these lesions may heal spontaneously or with special antibiotics, sometimes the bug can invade the joints and bones. As is the case with the vibrios, *Mycobacterium marinum* can be very severe in immunocompromised patients.

And of course there are the *Aeromonas* and *Plesiomonas* species. These organisms usually cause gastroenteritis, but both can lead to infection of the skin and other deeper tissues.

Why would a babysitter bathe a child before returning her to the parents?

"That may seem odd," says Mrs. Wolz, "but I have a really bad allergy to cats, and Marci keeps cats in the apartment too. That's why Marci generally sat for Katie at our house, but periodically, she'd take care of her at her apartment. On those occasions, I'd send a second outfit with Katie. Before I came to pick her up, Marci would bathe her and then dress her in the fresh clothes. The times we didn't do that, my nose would close right up because of the cat dander."

Two days later, the result from the piranha tank water was available: positive for PS. Tippen speculates that the dirty piranha water must have been emptied into the tub on one occasion just before Katie's bath. Some of the bacteria would have still been on the wet surface of the tub when Marci filled it up for Katie's bath. When Katie put the washcloth in her mouth, the PS got into her gastrointestinal tract. This was the last link in the chain of events that explained the strange case of Katie Wolz.

It was not the last step the epidemiologists took, however. The Missouri Department of Health launched an investigation to determine how commonly fish tanks were contaminated with PS. Public health agents sampled water from eighteen random aquariums at a number of pet shops and private homes across the state (including at least two tanks from each of Missouri's six regional health districts). To their surprise, they were able to isolate PS in four of the tanks, or 22 percent. Three different pet shops had water that tested positive. None of the fish in those tanks were sick, nor were any of the employees in the three pet shops that had positive results. To prevent disease in the employees, the Department of Health simply recommended that the employees wash their hands after contact with the aquarium water or the fish.

Marci and Kevin continued to keep piranhas, and Marci continued to care for little Katie. The solution to that problem also proved remarkably simple. Marci and Kevin continue to empty their fish tank in the tub, but they wash the tub with bleach afterward.

Katie recovered completely. Dr. Ramsey obtained two sets of follow-up surveillance cultures; both were negative, proving that Katie had completely eradicated the unusual bacteria from her body. She has remained well ever since.

~~~~~~~~~~

"We had recently returned from California when it all started," says Josephine Limone, thinking back to June 1992, when she got sick. "My husband Alfonso is a dentist, and we had just gone to a dental convention in Palm Springs. Several weeks after we returned, I remember that my underarms got very sore, first the left side I think and then the right. It was especially sore when I moved my arms. I took the subway to work and when I reached up to grab the handrail on the train, it really hurt."

Limone, an attractive woman with shoulder-length dark brown hair, was twenty-five at the time. She and Alfonso lived in midtown Manhattan, where she worked as an assistant administrator for the clinical laboratory at Mount Sinai Medical Center. "The next thing I noticed was swelling under my arms; it felt like marbles. Alfonso took a look and said they were swollen lymph glands. I was actually going to go to my gynecologist, because the location of one of them was closer to the breast tissue. That had me a little worried. The possibility of breast cancer did cross my mind."

But the next day, as she was dressing for work, Limone detected the strangest symptom of all—small blemishes had appeared on various parts of her body. "At first, I thought it was just acne," she recalls, "but they were in unusual locations: on my stomach, on my shins, one on my knee." She applied witch hazel to the pimples, hoping that they would dry up in a day or so. But a couple of days later they still had not cleared up, and then she began experiencing dull headaches and a low-grade fever. She knew it was time to see a doctor.

"I asked Dr. Neville Coleman, the medical director of the lab where I worked at the time, to take a look at the blemishes," Limone recalls. "He knew that I'd had chicken pox about a year before, and thought it might be a recurrence." So Coleman called to speak to Edward J. Bottone, Ph.D., a professor of medicine and microbiology at Mount Sinai. The two doctors briefly discussed the case, and Coleman sent Josephine up to Bottone's office for a formal consultation.

As part of his examination, Bottone carefully opened up one of Limone's whiteheads—tiny raised lesions filled with pus—and took a sample to examine under the microscope. He first applied special stains used to diagnose chicken pox, a viral disease. That test was normal, quickly ruling out that possibility. Using other stains, he also looked for bacteria. There were some white blood cells and a few slender rodlike bacteria. He carefully placed some of this material on a culture plate to determine what kind of bacteria, if any, were present. The culture would take a couple of days to get definitive results.

In the meantime, he told Limone to call him right away if she developed any new blemishes.

Diagnosing a patient with a rash is sometimes deceptively simple, and other times remarkably difficult. The cornerstone of any attempt at diagnosis is the patient's history. This starts with the most basic demographic facts: age, gender, ethnicity, occupation, recreational habits, and hobbies. The next phase is for the doctor to understand the course of events. Did the rash begin on one part of the skin and then spread to another, or did it begin all over the body at the same time? Does the patient have other associated symptoms? A fever or diarrhea, a swollen joint or a headache? Is the patient taking any new medications, whether prescribed by a doctor, over-the-counter, or herbal? Is there a pet in the house? Are there any allergies, either environmental or to medications? Does anyone else in the family have a similar eruption? What about coworkers?

There are countless potential questions, and as in any detective investigation, the answer to one question often suggests several new ones. If there is a pet in the house, what kind is it, and is it healthy? If other individuals in the same household are sick, did their symptoms begin at the same time or before or after? Was there any common exposure? If there is evolution of the rash, did it spread over hours, days, or weeks?

And as in any investigation, at least at the beginning, it may not be clear which line of inquiry will yield dividends and which will end in blind alleys. So the wise clinician starts out with as few preconceived notions as possible. At the beginning, one does not usually know which answers will, in the end, be the ones that lead to the correct diagnosis.

Although the history is most important, the physical examination is also important, especially in diagnosing patients with rash. Dermatologists describe different kinds of rashes. Is it flat or raised? If raised, is there any fluid in the bumps? And if there is fluid, is it clear fluid or pus? Doctors refer to these characteristics as the morphology of a rash, and while important, morphological distinctions are limited, since the skin has only so many ways it can manifest various disease states.

A flat spot is called a macule; a raised spot is called a papule. When a papule is filled with pus, it's called a pustule, and if it's filled with clear fluid it is a vesicle. The morphology of a rash helps, to some extent, limit the possible causes. The rash of Lyme disease, for example, is usually a very large macule. Chicken pox is generally vesicular.

Of course the distribution of a rash is also a very important clue to a diagnosis. Is the entire body covered with the rash? Are there spots separated by normal skin, or does one flow into the others to form a large confluent area of rash? The evolution of a rash can also be valuable evidence. In a patient with blisters, are all the blisters at the same stage, or have some scabbed over while new ones are still forming in other areas of the skin?

These are some of the cases where diagnosing a rash can be deceptively simple; it is a matter of pattern recognition. The doctor will take one look and make a pronouncement with authority. A rash on one wrist may result from contact dermatitis, a reaction to something in a watchband. An eruption localized along a well-defined strip of skin (called a dermatome, an area associated with a given cutaneous nerve) is likely due to shingles, which is caused by a recrudescence of the chicken-pox virus in a particular spinal nerve.

A few days later, Limone did return, with a new pimple on her upper right arm. "I did two things," recalls Bottone. "I asked her to see an infectious diseases specialist. He thought it was possible that the rash was something she may have contracted from an insect bite but was not impressed by the lesion. Then I referred her to a dermatologist, Dr. Marsha Gordon."

Dr. Gordon had seen Limone a few times in the past for minor problems, including her recent case of chicken pox. After taking a look, she brought in a second dermatologist to examine the patient. "They asked me all the usual questions about whether I had used any new soaps, new detergents, that sort of thing," says Limone. The doctors told her that they thought she had some sort of viral infection of the skin. This usually means that a person has a virus in the body that is showing itself in the form of skin lesions. The common childhood diseases—measles, German measles, and chicken pox—are typical examples.

Dr. Gordon's handwritten office note dated June 25, 1992, reads, "Patient developed bilateral axillary lymphadenopathy 5 days ago and 4 days ago, began developing evanescent pustules—few scattered . . . presently only one pustule on right arm. Several scattered red papules (status post pustules). The oral mucosa is clear. There is increased axillary lymph nodes (no groin nodes)."

But the doctors needed to do more tests before they could provide a definitive diagnosis. It was at this point, Limone remembers, that she began to grow more concerned. She never imagined that her condition was anything out of the ordinary. "Physically, I didn't feel that sick," she says. "But I was really worried that no one could tell me what was causing my symptoms."

Gordon admits she was a bit puzzled. Based on Limone's medical history and the fact that her lesions did not fit the patterns of various other infections, the dermatologist was able to rule out the most common causes of such symptoms: shingles, herpes simplex (the virus that causes cold sores, which can sometimes spread throughout the body), and contact dermatitis—a rash or other allergic reaction that occurs when the skin touches an irritant. Because the morphology of the lesions was pustular, the possibility of a sexually transmitted disease—disseminated gonorrhea—was also raised, but for all sorts of clinical and epidemiological reasons, this diagnosis was immediately discarded.

The dermatologist thought that a nonspecific viral cause was most likely, but was waiting anxiously to see the results of the culture that Bottone had taken, because there was one other possibility that the doctors were considering.

So Gordon was relieved when the lab report showed a crucial piece of information that would help narrow the search. The tests that Bottone had done on samples from Limone's lesions turned out to be positive for a rather unusual bacterium called *Pseudomonas aeruginosa*, which we will call PA. At least now the doctors knew what was causing Limone's symptoms. But having this particular label offered little solace.

The pseudomonas is a large group of bacteria; there are hundreds of individual strains. They were first described in 1894. Most are completely harmless and do not cause disease in humans. *Pseudomonas aeruginosa* is an extremely hardy bacterium that can grow under almost any conditions, as long as there's moisture. The bug is commonly found in soil, water, and on the surface of plants and animals.

Its nutritional requirements are extremely basic, which allows it to grow just about anywhere. The bug produces two types of soluble pigments: the fluorescent pigment pyoverdin and the blue pigment pyocyanin. The blue pigment functions in iron metabolism in the bacterium. It is also responsible for the so-called "blue pus" that is a characteristic of PA infections.

The PA bug especially loves swimming pools, and because it grows over a wide temperature range, it will also lurk in whirlpools and hot tubs that have not been properly disinfected with chlorine. Healthy people don't normally get PA infections; it's more common in those whose immune symptoms have been weakened by chemotherapy or a serious illness or other infection. PA is called an "opportunistic" bacterium. This means that, although it does not normally infect humans, when given the chance it will strike and often with a vengeance.

It causes severe, often fatal infections in patients whose normal host defense mechanisms are compromised. Patients with burns, cancer, AIDS, diabetes, and cystic fibrosis are particularly vulnerable. Once inside the body, the bacteria can cause severe infections of the bloodstream, heart, lungs, urinary tract, skin, eye, external ear canal, bones, and joints.

Even though it is rare, PA can occasionally cause infections in healthy individuals. Given its proclivity for moist environments, it can often be cultured out of tennis shoes, and if a person steps on a nail while wearing a shoe, the PA is often inoculated into the foot and can cause a serious bone or joint infection. Another condition sometimes reported in non-immunocompromised people is a skin infection called folliculitis (an infection of the hair follicles).

Folliculitis from PA was already a well-known entity in 1992. In the mid-1970s, articles began to surface that described people developing PA skin infections after bathing in whirlpool tubs. One of the first was a paper published in the *Journal of the American Medical Association* that documented thirty-two individuals who developed generalized pustular rash after using a particular whirlpool in Minnesota in March 1975. The attack rate was over 50 percent, since sixty-one people had been exposed. The rash appeared in as few as eight hours to as late as two days after exposure and resolved within seven days. None of the thirty-seven motel guests who did not use the pool developed the rash. The same strain of the bacterium PA was isolated from the skin lesions of some of the patients as well as from the water. The authors concluded: "Circumstantial evidence implicated the whirlpool as the most probable source of infection. Deficiencies in disinfecting equipment and technique were identified and corrected."

Numerous other reports followed. The common denominator seemed to be heavy usage of a hot tub or exposure toward the end of a day (suggesting that the number of humans in the tub, or "bather density," was an important factor) and time spent in the tub. The degree of chlorination was also an issue, as was the temperature. The incubation period in all these early studies was usually no longer than forty-eight hours, and all cases resolved. There were some reports of people becoming infected in home hot tubs, and others documented infections that were not limited to the skin. Patients developed pneumonia, urinary tract infections, and keratitis (infection of the cornea) after hot tub exposures.

In 1980, doctors in Tennessee reported a slightly larger outbreak, this one related to exposure to an indoor swimming pool at a health club. The first hint of a problem was in November, when a local physician reported the occurrence of unusual skin lesions in three patients whose only common link was membership in a health club. A culture done on one of the patients grew out PA. The CDC was called in to investigate, and the inquiry uncovered a total of thirty-seven members who developed a pustular rash that had started hours to days after use of the swimming pool. Another ten patrons had symptoms of an external ear infection also thought to be part of the outbreak, but without any skin involvement.

A month before the outbreak, the club had installed a new indoor heated swimming pool with an automatic filter and chlorinator. On Wednesday, November 5, the managers noticed that the pool water was turbid. When they checked the chlorinator, they discovered that it was broken. The pH of the water was higher than it should have been, and they could not detect any free chlorine. But while they made the necessary repairs, they kept the pool open to the members.

The investigators found that, as is typical for PA, only hair-bearing skin was involved (as would be expected from a folliculitis). The palms of the hands, soles of the feet, and mucous membranes were never involved. There was a predilection for the buttocks, axilla, and trunk, but not typically the arms and legs. Many patients had low-grade fever or a feeling of malaise. All of the patients had normal immune systems, and they all got better without any serious consequences.

The authors of the Tennessee study also focused on forestalling further outbreaks, concluding: "Prevention of pseudomonas folliculitis should be possible by maintenance of pool water at a pH of 7.2–7.8, and free available chlorine levels at > 0.5 mg/liter. Swimming pools usually are maintained within these limits, which may explain why outbreaks associated with them are rare. It is more difficult to maintain adequate pH and chlorine levels in heated whirlpools and baths because their heavier load of bathers per volume of water creates a greater demand for chlorine, and their higher temperatures and agitation cause an increase in loss of chlorine into the air."

Three years later, in 1983, the CDC reported an even larger epidemic, this one associated with use of a waterslide in Utah. The first patients developed symptoms on the evening of April 30. On May 3, the Salt Lake City-County Health Department notified state authorities that people were developing skin rashes and earaches after using a long curved slide that empties into a pool. By May 7, just four days later, 265 cases had been identified. The investigators sent out questionnaires to more than 200 people from two church groups that had visited the facility on April 30. Of people who went on the waterslide, 76 percent got sick, but none of the unexposed visitors developed symptoms.

Of those who did fall ill, over 90 percent had the characteristic skin lesions. Nearly half had headaches and a quarter had fever. In a particularly unusual case, one patient had a temperature of 104 degrees and needed to be hospitalized.

For patients who already suffer from a serious illness, exposure to PA can have quite different outcomes, as is seen from a small outbreak in a major Iowa hospital. Over a fourteen-month period, seven patients, all of whom had forms of leukemia, were diagnosed with PA infection, which came from the drain of a whirlpool bath in the hospital's oncology unit. Four of the seven died.

Armed with the positive PA culture, and knowing the organism's predilection for water, Bottone focused his next round of questions for Limone on various aquatic exposures. If the infection had started during the trip to California, the incubation period would be exceptionally long. But this is where Bottone's started.

"When the culture turned positive for PA, Dr. Bottone asked me all sorts of other questions," Limone recalls. "Because of my California trip, he had me retracing my steps, verifying that I hadn't gone into a sauna or a hot tub.

"Then he asked me to think about my daily routine; he really got into the nitty-gritty," says Limone. "It was a bit embarrassing because we had a strictly professional relationship, so it was a little out of place. But he was now in the capacity of the clinician and I tried to view him that way. He had lots of questions.

"Did my husband use the same washcloth as I did? The same bar of soap? How many showers did I take? When did I shave? What lotions and creams did I use? I had to bring all my toiletries to the lab. He took cultures of my soap, baby lotion, moisturizing cream, and shaving cream, thinking that one of them might be contaminated with the bacteria."

But they weren't.

Still, Bottone was convinced that Limone must have come in contact with something harboring PA. "Knowing that the normal habitat of this organism is moisture, I persisted," Bottone recalls. "I asked her how she took showers. When I asked about the washcloth, she said, 'No, I use a loofah sponge.' At the time, I had no idea what a loofah sponge was, so I asked to see it."

Something clicked when Bottone saw the loofah. "Josephine brought this big sponge in," he recalls. "It was still a little wet, and when you squeezed it, a small bit of water with a greenish tint dripped out." Dr. Bottone was well aware of the pigments that PA forms—pyoverdin and pyocyanin. The green liquid that oozed out of the loofah was clearly consistent with those pigments. Figuring it was some kind of bacteria, he had the sponge tested. It was loaded with PA.

Although they look like something that might come out of the sea, loofah sponges (or luffa as they are sometimes called) are actually made from the gourdlike fruit of a tropical and subtropical vine called *Luffa*, a genus that includes six species. The ripe fruit resembles a large cucumber, which is not surprising because the plant belongs to the Cucurbitaceae family, which also includes cucumbers, squashes, gourds, and melons.

The vines are traditionally cultivated in India and the Middle East, where the name originates, and are also grown in other warm, dry regions. Loofah is harvested for food in many parts of Asia. All species are edible if the loofah fruits are cooked and eaten before they mature; otherwise, they are too tough to eat. Loofah sometimes appears on menus as Chinese okra.

The loofah is the only plant source of sponges, which have been used in kitchens and bathhouses for centuries. When grown to make sponges, the loofah fruit is allowed to mature and dry on the vine. The woody exterior skin is peeled away, and the seeds are shaken out for replanting. The drying process leaves behind only the network of xylem, which is the tubular transport system used to carry nutrients from one part of the plant to another. This dense web of straw-colored fibers will puff up again once the loofah is moistened.

The resulting sponge is most commonly used in place of a washcloth in the shower. Many people prefer to use the loofah as a dry exfoliating brush before bathing, which gently removes the surface layer of dead skin and leaves the skin smooth and conditioned. In the kitchen, the loofah's coarse texture makes it great for cleaning dishes and countertops, but it is gentle enough for use on delicate items like coated cookware that could be damaged by normal abrasives. Like other sponges, loofah will collect bacteria if it is kept moist and warm, and because they are made from a living organism, loofah sponges can hold bacteria more easily than synthetic fibers.

But how, Bottone wondered, did the bacteria get there in the first place? Unfortunately, he wasn't able to come up with any definitive answer. He did prove that the PA strain in the sponge was the same one that he had cultured from Limone's skin lesion. It was the exact same serotype, so it was certain that the loofah had infected Limone.

Bottone theorized that Limone might have picked up the PA at work in the hospital lab. But he excluded this as a likely possibility for two reasons. For one, Limone worked in an administrative area, not a clinical one. Also, Bottone collected and cultured the loofahs of ten different microbiology technicians and found that none of them were positive for PA.

His other theory was that trace amounts of PA in her home's running water contaminated Limone's sponge and then grew freely when the sponge was kept wet. Small amounts of PA are occasionally found in water supplies, even in tap water. The number of organisms is small, however, and not harmful (even if we drink the water, the tiny portion of bacteria is killed by our stomach acid before it can hurt us). But it can lead to problems if it's allowed to grow.

Limone took two showers daily, and her husband (who didn't use the sponge) took one every day. Limone kept the loofah, which measured four by eight inches, hanging on the hot water knob in the shower. Because of the sponge's size, where she kept it, and the number of showers it was exposed to each day, it never dried out enough for the bacteria to die. When she showered with the contaminated loofah, she was essentially rubbing the bacteria all over her skin, inoculating herself through tiny cuts from shaving her legs or perhaps even through minor skin abrasions caused by the loofah itself.

Bottone tested individual pieces of loofah. He found that when he placed very small quantities of PA onto a loofah and let it sit overnight, the number of organisms the next morning had multiplied over a thousandfold. Other experiments showed that loofahs incubated with tap water or even distilled water would also start growing PA.

Doctors say that any sponge—or even a washcloth—that remains wet all the time is prone to harbor bacteria. People typically launder their washcloths periodically, which removes the bacteria, but they usually don't put their sponges in the washing machine. So sponges are far more likely to be the culprit. Sponges made from natural materials (such as loofah or sea sponges) are most susceptible to contamination.

After solving Josephine Limone's medical mystery, Edward Bottone went in search of ways to make natural sponges safer to use. He found that soaking a sponge in a 10 percent solution of household bleach (one part bleach to nine parts water) for about five minutes, then thoroughly rinsing, was very effective against bacteria. The sponges should be soaked at least once a week.

One microbiologist, Dr. George Tortora from the State University of New York at Stony Brook, experimented with using a microwave oven to sterilize sponges and loofahs. He found that microwaving them for two minutes on the high setting would kill nearly all the bugs, and five minutes would completely sterilize the sponges. He cautions that the sponge must be wet when microwaved, because the high temperature of the resultant steam is what sterilizes it.

Shortly after Bottone's case report appeared in the medical literature, another instance appeared, but this one was related to a synthetic sponge made of nonwoven polyester. The case was almost a carbon copy of Limone's: a healthy thirty-two-year-old woman developed forty to fifty papules on all parts of her body over a four-day period. A culture of one of the skin lesions was positive for PA. She had no exposures to hot tubs or swimming pools. Her doctor cultured her sponge and found the same organism.

Another case report described an almost identical situation, but this time the offending vector for the PA was a Caribbean sea sponge that a forty-four-year-old woman was using in the shower.

Shortly thereafter, Italian physicians reported on fourteen patients who had acquired PA folliculitis from their home showers. All had typical patterns of pustular rashes that grew out PA on culture. In five families, two or more members had the disease at the same time. The investigators found that the sources of the PA included well water, the filter from a washing machine, a bidet, and the bathroom sink faucet.

In another strange but related outbreak, in April 2002, a cardboard box manufacturing plant in Arkansas hired an environmental health consultant to look into a cluster of employees who had been plagued by unusual skin rashes. It turned out that the facility had recently switched to a closed system for the water used in its industrial process, wherein the used water is recycled and treated and then reused by the box-making machinery. Twenty-seven employees had pustular rashes on their arms, legs, and torsos. The recycled water grew out PA.

The closed recycling system was abandoned, and the pipes were thoroughly cleaned. The employees were educated about the source of the rashes, and hand-washing stations were created. Glove use was also encouraged. Follow-up surveillance showed no more PA in the water, and the employees remained healthy.

Two different groups of physicians, one from southern France and the other in Pennsylvania, described a total of four other unusual cases of PA skin infection that was related to wetsuit use by scuba divers. All of these case reports and clusters of cases show just how ubiquitous PA is. After all, water is everywhere.

Once Bottone had figured out the cause of Limone's strange malady, curing it was simple. She took an antibiotic, and within a couple of weeks she was fully recovered. Even the pimples disappeared completely. Still, the experience changed at least one aspect of Limone's life: she's sworn off loofah sponges forever. "I never use them anymore at all," she says. "In fact, I'm even cautious about using a washcloth.

"A lot of my friends buy at the Body Shop, and they make these gift baskets with bath oil beads and the loofah sponges. I always tell everyone the story. I think people can relate to it because they all use them too."

~~~~~~~~~~~~~~~~

It began as innocently as a thousand other cases. It could have happened anywhere, and it might have involved any family. So on the evening of Sunday, November 10, 1991, Peter and Michele Burdick were not particularly alarmed when their only child, Emily—a petite blonde, not quite four years old at the time—began having abdominal cramps and diarrhea. Such symptoms are a normal part of growing up, and nearly every child at some point will have them. When Michele began to feel some cramps too, she figured that it was just something that they had both eaten.

"The next morning, Emily woke me up early, complaining of a stomach ache. I told her to lie down and that it would probably go away," recalls Michele, who is from Somerset, Massachusetts, "but by afternoon, it hadn't gone away; in fact, she was worse. That evening I noticed some blood in her stools." Monday was Veteran's Day, and the pediatrician's office closed early. Figuring that Emily would probably get better on her own, Michele waited until Tuesday to bring her daughter to the doctor. Dr. Margaret Bello, covering for Emily's regular pediatrician (Dr. Walter Rok), examined her and then arranged for blood tests and x-rays to be performed at St. Anne's Hospital in Fall River.

"This was Emily's first experience going through these kinds of tests. She was complaining that her tummy hurt and that she wanted to be carried," her mother recalled. After the tests were completed, the Burdicks returned home and arranged a follow-up visit for the next day. There was an implicit expectation that, as in most cases of diarrhea, mother's and daughter's symptoms would both start to resolve on their own.

But instead of turning the corner and improving, the situation deteriorated; Michele and Emily kept getting sicker.

"By late Tuesday, I developed cramps that seemed to worsen by the hour. Emily's trips to the bathroom were becoming more frequent. She was crying a lot and asking me to sit with her in the bathroom to rest her head on my lap. And my husband, Peter, was working the night shift from 6:30 PM to 6:30 AM, so I was all alone with Emily. Then I developed diarrhea and the cramps got much worse. It got to the point where I could barely assist Emily, my pains were so severe."

Peter called to check on his wife and daughter from his job on an assembly line at a nearly manufacturing mill. The report he received was not good. Emily and Michele spent the night on the couch because it was closer to the bathroom. But neither of them slept. As dawn approached, the situation turned far more ominous. Each bowel movement Michele had was progressively bloodier. Enough of toughing it out at home; they called the doctor back.

Dehydrated and now losing blood, both mother and daughter were promptly admitted to St. Anne's Hospital on Wednesday morning. Michele required intravenous fluids and pain killers. She was exhausted.

So was Peter. "I had been up all night at work," he remembers, "and felt stressed and anxious because Michele and Emily were so sick. It all happened so fast. On top of everything, we had previously scheduled a repair man to install a new stove that morning." He stayed with Emily in her hospital room all that day and night until his parents were able to come from Cape Cod to relieve him so he could get a few hours sleep. Thursday brought more of the same.

Emily and Michele Burdick were both suffering from gastroenteritis, the medical term for inflammation of the intestines. The most common symptoms are abdominal cramps, nausea, vomiting, and diarrhea. Even without blood, the volume of diarrhea can be so great that patients become seriously dehydrated. Worldwide, gastroenteritis is one of the most common diseases in humans. Infectious agents, mostly viruses and bacteria, are the usual culprits, but various toxins that these organisms produce, as well as some parasites and toxins from other sources, also cause gastroenteritis. Most cases are self-limited; even most cases of the bacterial variety resolve after a few days. The treatment is merely to replenish the body orally with fluids to prevent dehydration, and maybe take some acetaminophen or ibuprofen for the aches, pains, and fevers.

In spite of the simple treatment, gastroenteritis and dehydration are huge problems in the developing world. Childhood diarrhea is a common cause of mortality in the third world, where it accounts for 70 percent of all hospital admissions due to infectious diseases, as well as half of all childhood deaths in both India and Afghanistan. Cholera is one cause of gastroenteritis that, in the days before intensive rehydration therapies, had a very high death rate. But even viral gastroenteritis can kill an infant or small toddler pretty quickly, because they don't have large reserves of fluid in their little bodies. The loss of relatively small amounts of fluid leads to dehydration, which in severe cases can lead to death.

Replacing the fluids to prevent this outcome has traditionally needed to be done intravenously, but in recent decades doctors are increasingly using newly developed oral rehydration techniques, which are both very inexpensive and very effective, to reduce infant mortality in the third world.

When the diarrhea turns bloody, it generally means that the causative organism is bacterial or that there is some form of inflammatory condition of the colon, such as ulcerative colitis. In the first case, it suggests that the responsible organism is actually invading the wall of the intestine. Whatever the cause, the development of blood in the diarrhea is not a good thing, and can understandably frighten a patient, especially a child. Patients with bloody diarrhea sometimes lose enough blood to require a transfusion. But there are other, more sinister problems that may occur that have nothing to do with blood loss.

In Emily's case, soon after she was admitted to the hospital Dr. Rok took over her care. "The blood loss was substantial, and the initial stool cultures ruled out salmonella, shigella, and campylobacter—the more common causes of bloody diarrhea," he explained. On Friday, Dr. Rok received some alarming news from the lab: Emily's kidneys were shutting down.

The kidneys are two bean-shaped organs that lie deep in the abdomen. The heart pumps roughly 25 percent of the body's blood flow through the kidneys, which filter the blood to remove waste products. These wastes are then carried from the body through excretion in the urine.

Among the various substances the kidneys remove are two called urea nitrogen and creatinine. The level of urea nitrogen in the blood is abbreviated in medical lexicon as BUN (blood urea nitrogen). Measuring these two blood levels—the BUN and creatinine—is something that doctors across the country perform routinely millions of times each year to monitor their patients' kidney function. The normal level for BUN is less than 20 milligrams per deciliter, and for creatinine, less than about 1.2. When the BUN and creatinine levels rise above these values, the condition is known as renal insufficiency or kidney failure. There are different degrees of renal failure, and many different causes. So when they are faced with this situation, doctors go through a checklist to determine the reason. There are three general reasons for kidney failure. The first is called "pre-renal," meaning there is a problem in the system before blood reaches the kidneys. This usually means that not enough blood is getting to the kidneys, sometimes from very low blood pressure or severe dehydration. A certain amount of pressure is necessary for the kidneys to properly do their work, and if that blood pressure falls, the kidneys begin to fail and the levels of BUN and creatinine start to increase.

In another type of kidney failure, termed post-renal, the cause is a blockage or obstruction in one of the tubes that carry the urine from the kidneys out of the body. This is essentially a plumbing problem, and when the blockage is relieved, the kidney function usually promptly normalizes, and the levels of BUN and creatinine return to normal. One of the most common causes is obstruction of the flow of urine due to an enlarged prostate gland. In both pre-renal and post-renal failure, the kidneys themselves are not the source of the problem.

The third kind of renal failure is when the kidneys themselves do not function correctly; the problem is intrinsic to the kidneys themselves. The list of possible causes of this kind of renal failure is long and includes problems due to immunological attack, infection, side effects from various medications, and a host of others. An example of immunological attack is called glomerulonephritis. There are many causes of this condition, one of which is the after effects of strep throat. Over time, chronic medical conditions such as high blood pressure and diabetes can lead to intrinsic renal failure.

The treatment of a patient with renal failure will depend entirely on the cause. If it is due to severe dehydration leading to pre-renal failure, intravenous fluids will often do the trick. In most cases of post-renal problems, the solution is mechanical. If there is trouble with the prostate, doctors will insert a small catheter into the bladder to relieve the obstruction of urine. Some cases of renal failure resulting from intrinsic kidney disease are treated with steroids; others require more powerful immune modulating drugs. But if these treatments do not work, intrinsic renal failure may require treatment with an "artificial kidney," known as a dialysis machine.

When Dr. Rok saw that Emily's BUN was 35 and her creatinine was 2.6, he quickly sought to determine the specific cause. There were two clues that led Dr. Rok to consider the possibility of a most unusual disease. One hint was the appearance of Emily's red blood cells under a microscope: the cells appeared shredded, ripped apart, or hemolyzed, in medical jargon. The second was the context in which the kidney failure was occurring: bloody diarrhea. Although he had seen only one case, years ago when he was in training, Dr. Rok was pretty sure that he was dealing with a case of hemolytic uremic syndrome, or HUS.

First described in 1955, HUS is a rare disease. The medical term for kidney failure is uremia, and the condition that causes the shredded cells that Dr. Rok saw under the microscope is hemolysis—hence the term hemolytic uremic syndrome. Experts believe that the symptoms result from damage to the lining of small blood vessels in the kidney, which leads to the renal failure. Blood platelets, an essential component of normal blood clotting, drop to precariously low levels. The kidneys and blood cells are not the only organs that can be affected: sometimes the liver becomes involved. Occasionally patients develop neurological symptoms, such as seizures and coma. More ominously, in approximately 5 percent of patients with HUS, the outcome is fatal.

For many years, the cause of HUS was unclear. Instances would occur sporadically in various locations. Some of these cases were associated with infections of different kinds, often intestinal infections, such as gastroenteritis.

Most cases are associated with eating food that has been contaminated with *Escherichia coli* bacteria. *E. coli* is an extraordinarily common bug that is present in enormous quantities in the intestinal tracts of humans and other mammals. It was first described in 1885 by a German pediatrician and microbiologist named Theodor Escherich, for whom it is named—the colon bacillus of Escherich. In humans, these bacteria colonize an infant's intestine within the first two days of life.

There are hundreds of different kinds of E. coli; each of these variations is called a serotype, and they are distinguished by a particular protein signature. Microbiologists describe the various types of E. coli by categorizing the proteins on the bacteria. On the body of the bug, there are proteins designated as "O," and on the flagella (the whiplike arms the bacterium uses for locomotion), there are "H" proteins, and so forth.

In December 1981, an outbreak of bloody diarrhea occurred in Medford, Oregon, and one of its suburbs, White City. Medford is a medium-sized town located in the Rogue Valley, west of the Cascade Mountain range. The tests for the standard pathogens that cause bloody diarrhea were negative, and the Oregon public health officials could not come up with an answer. They requested assistance from the CDC in Atlanta, which promptly dispatched a team of investigators. The lead investigator was a young epidemiology intelligence officer, Lee W. Riley, who flew out to Oregon the next day. The investigators were able to culture an extremely rare form of E. coli from most of the affected patients. When the protein tests were done, the strain was given the rather unceremonious name of O157:H7. At that time, E. coli bacteria were not thought to cause diarrhea, and because it is so common in human feces, nobody initially thought it was significant.

The following May, as the Oregon investigation was unfolding, another cluster of patients with bloody diarrhea was identified in Traverse City, Michigan. The same O157:H7 strain was identified. The common denominator in both outbreaks was eating hamburgers from McDonald's fast food outlets. When the CDC searched its database of more than three thousand E. coli samples, there was only a single specimen that matched the strain from the Oregon and Michigan outbreaks. It was from a stool sample of a fifty-year-old female naval officer from Oakland, California, and it had been collected in 1975. When the Navy dug up her records, it was found that she had been sick with a case of bloody diarrhea.

As Riley and his team traced the meat back from McDonald's, they found that one of the restaurant's suppliers, a plant in Ohio, had saved some of the ground beef, ironically, as part of a quality control program. The same *E. coli* O157:H7 strain was found in that sample, which was from the same lot that ended up in the hamburgers the patients had eaten. This was groundbreaking science, although none of the patients from these two outbreaks developed HUS.

This is where the work of Canadian researchers comes into the story. Dr. Mohamed Karmali, a microbiologist, was trying to put other pieces of this same puzzle together. In the summer of 1980, within a ten-day period, fourteen Toronto-area children were diagnosed with HUS—an extraordinary number of cases of such a rare disease in so short a time. Aware of the recent work by another Canadian microbiologist who had described a toxin in some *E. coli* that could play a role, Karmali tested these children for the presence of this toxin in *E. coli*, and he found it. Expanding the scope of his investigation, in 1985, he reported results of forty children with HUS and found evidence for this new toxin in most of them. He concluded, "Our findings indicate that [toxin-producing] *E. coli* have a close, and probably causal association with idiopathic HUS of childhood."

These outbreaks, especially because they were associated with such a prominent company as McDonald's, hit the national press and were featured in large newspaper headlines. Some referred to it as "hamburger disease." McDonald's stock took a temporary hit, but it soon rebounded. Americans' consciousness about developing HUS from eating hamburgers increased as well.

The problem surfaced again in 1993 (two years after Emily's case), once more raising HUS to national prominence when a large number of children in the Seattle area became sick after eating hamburgers from a Jack-in-the-Box restaurant. The outbreak came to light in January, when the Washington Department of Health was notified of a cluster of children with bloody diarrhea, and HUS was noticed in Seattle-area hospitals. In that epidemic, 602 patients developed bloody diarrhea or HUS, of which 477 had culture-confirmed *E. coli* infection.

This outbreak was tightly clustered in time, with a peak incidence of illness between January 17 and 20; 144 patients required hospitalization, and 30 developed HUS. Three children died from the kidney disease.

Investigators tracing the sources of the hamburger meat found that 73 Jack-in-the-Box restaurants were responsible; the beef had ultimately come from five slaughter plants in the United States and another one in Canada.

In the aftermath of litigation that resulted from the epidemic, company officials admitted that they had been warned by local health departments that their hamburgers must be cooked to an internal temperature of 155 degrees Fahrenheit; however, they felt that this "overcooking" led to the meat having a tough texture. Numerous class-action and individual lawsuits were settled for many tens of millions of dollars.

Emily's case happened between these two large outbreaks. During this period, HUS had become one of the most common causes of intrinsic renal failure in children in the United States. For a specialist in childhood kidney disease, this is a relatively common problem, but it's not one that most general pediatricians see with any frequency. One mark of a great doctor is the ability to know when to ask for help. Dr. Rok knew that his next move was clear: Emily would have to be transferred to a hospital in Boston where pediatric kidney specialists and dialysis facilities were available.

"I was very worried about Emily, and I felt helpless in being able to be with her during the most frightening part of her illness," remembers Michele, who was still having copious bloody stools and was tethered to an IV line. On the Friday after she got sick, Emily and her dad traveled by ambulance to Children's Hospital in Boston. Her kidney function was failing. At the hospital, Emily had a catheter inserted in her bladder to measure her urine output, and she was put on intravenous fluids.

The following day was one of the hardest for her father. "I don't know which was worse," Peter recalls. "Michele was still hospitalized and couldn't be with us and Emily had to go the operating room to have a dialysis catheter placed just below her collarbone. It was all beginning to hit me." Except for when she was in the operating room, Peter didn't let Emily out of his sight for the next five days.

As remarkable and unfortunate as Emily's situation had become, it was made all the more extraordinary by events that were still unfolding back in Fall River. Dr. Rok had a second patient hospitalized at St.

Anne's. She was Margaret Carvalho, a vibrant twenty-two-month-old toddler with short light brown hair whose case seemed to be a carbon copy of Emily's: bloody diarrhea followed by dehydration and then listless behavior. Margaret was hospitalized on Thursday, November 14. By Sunday, three days later, her kidneys were also beginning to fail.

"So I was back on the phone to Boston," recalls Dr. Rok, who, after not seeing a single case of HUS in his twelve years of practice, felt pretty sure that he was now dealing with his second case in as many days.

The specialist at Children's Hospital was Dr. Melanie Kim, director of the general renal program. On Wednesday, November 20, two more girls—sisters, and patients of another Fall River pediatrician—were transferred to Children's Hospital with HUS. "This was very unusual," recalls Dr. Kim, who, as a specialist at a regional referral center, generally sees about twelve cases of HUS each year, usually clustered around June and July. "So to see four cases from the same small town in November was quite striking. We notified the state Department of Public Health." Besides the four girls from Fall River, there were already two children in Dr. Kim's unit with HUS, one from northern New England and another from Boston.

By this time, a key piece of information had emerged: stool cultures from three of the Fall River girls (including Emily and Margaret) turned positive for the *E. coli* serotype O157:H7 bacteria. It was happening again.

Dr. Susan Lett is the director of epidemiology at the Department of Public Health in Massachusetts. "Knowing the relationship between *E. coli* diarrhea and HUS, we decided to investigate. I contacted the CDC in Atlanta for help."

Dr. Richard Besser was a pediatrician with the CDC's Epidemiology Intelligence Service. "I had signed up with the enteric [intestinal] diseases branch because I thought I'd be on the road a lot working on various disease outbreaks. As it turned out, I had been doing desk work and fielding routine telephone calls that get directed to our branch. Being in Atlanta four months without an outbreak to investigate, I was a little stir crazy."

After receiving the call from Dr. Lett in Boston, Dr. Besser's supervisor directed him to fly to Boston the next day. "I was champing at the bit," recalls Dr. Besser. "I was very excited!" On Friday, November 22, he took the short flight to Boston. The next morning, he and Dr. Lett began the investigation. That weekend, they interviewed the families, spending several hours with each one. Dr. Besser recalls that "the families had already arrived at the tentative conclusion relating the illnesses to a frozen fish product. In fact, when we arrived at the hospital, people asked us if we were there to investigate the fish stick outbreak."

The epidemiologists launched a three-pronged investigation. The first task was to identify any other cases involved in the outbreak. Dr. Lett's office sent out notices to area pediatricians, family practitioners, and medical laboratories. Simultaneously, Lett and Besser spent most of the first few days exhaustively interviewing the families to try to find the common denominator in the case. What had infected them with the *E. coli* 0157:H7? And last, the third prong of attack, the investigators sent the bacteria isolated from each child to the lab to see if they were identical.

This last strategy proved very helpful, because the DNA fingerprint of the bacteria from one of the children who was not from the Fall River area was different from the DNA fingerprint of the bacteria from the four local girls. "That limited the scope of our investigation," said Dr. Besser.

The epidemiologists spent hours trying to pinpoint a common food that all the patients had eaten so they might identify the source. The families all shopped at the same store, and of course there was the fish stick theory—which was quickly put to rest. Fish sticks from the store where they had been purchased, as well as some of the original fish sticks still in the families' freezers, did not contain the bacteria. Hamburgers were another obvious possibility. After cataloguing everything the patients had eaten and drunk, the investigators interviewed neighbors who were not sick. Epidemiologists call this a case-control study, an attempt to see if there were any differences in the diets of those neighbors who did get sick compared with those who did not.

From the case-control studies, recalls Dr. Lett, "there were no obvious high-risk foods—chicken or hamburger—and we had checked the fish sticks." This was odd: most previous outbreaks had been linked to ground beef. The investigators were beginning to get discouraged, but using computer software to analyze the data, a most unusual and unexpected trend emerged. The patients were far more likely than their healthy neighbors to have drunk apple cider.

While the epidemiologists were busy collecting their information, Emily Burdick was getting sicker; her kidneys had deteriorated to the point that she needed dialysis. After the dialysis catheter was placed, she developed a fever and had to be watched in the ICU for a day and a half. There she received her first dialysis treatment. This involves pumping the patient's blood out through a catheter and into a dialysis machine— an artificial kidney—which removes the waste products. Then the purified blood is pumped back into the body. Even for an adult, this treatment is not very easy to tolerate.

"Emily had to lie very still in an uncomfortable position for the dialysis," remembers her father, "and the main thing she hated was when the bandage covering the catheter was removed. It hurt. We bought her a puppet—Clifford the red dog—and that was a help; Clifford occasionally got a laugh out of Emily." Everything that happened to Emily also happened to Clifford: blood drawing, blood pressure monitoring, and bandage changes.

To reduce the frequency of the ninety-minute dialysis treatments, Emily's fluid intake was severely restricted, so that her body wouldn't swell between sessions. "Anyone who has lived with a four year-old knows how little they like to brush their teeth, but Emily constantly asked me if she could brush her teeth, because she would suck up the water from the bristles of the toothbrush, she was so thirsty," recalls Michele, who had improved enough to be discharged from the hospital and was spending all her time with Emily.

She remembers going to dialysis with Emily and seeing outpatients coming in for their treatments, and wondering if Emily would need long-term dialysis. The families from Fall River shared the anxiety of having a seriously ill child in the hospital. "One of the children with HUS not from our area had neurological symptoms. He couldn't walk, and when he was discharged, it was to a rehab facility. It was then that we realized that it could get a lot worse," remembers Michele. "We also gave each other encouragement when any of the girls showed signs of improvement."

The advisories that had been sent out to local doctors led to the identification of eighteen cases of the *E. coli* diarrhea, and ultimately the tally rose to twenty-three. After apple cider became the prime suspect, Besser and Lett went back to the parents to find out where they had bought their cider. The majority remembered buying it locally at the Old Swanzey Orchard. Old Swanzey, whose main business is garden equipment and nursery supplies, is housed in a large red barn-like structure. Behind that is a smaller red shed that houses a traditional wood cider press. During the fall, the proprietor would make one or two batches of fresh cider every week.

Apple cider is a raw, unprocessed product. The apples are ground into a pulp called pomace, which is then put into a mesh held in place by a wooden frame. The hydraulic press squeezes the pomace and the cider trickles out. It is neither filtered nor pasteurized; if you look at the bottom of a bottle of cider, you will see the sediment. Cider is a natural product that will ferment, or harden, even when refrigerated. It is different from apple juice, which is filtered and pasteurized to sterilize the product.

The association of apple cider with disease was a surprise to the investigators because it's a very acidic beverage—it is generally thought to be too acidic to support the growth of bacteria. But when Dr. Besser reviewed the medical literature, he found a precedent: a 1980 outbreak of HUS in Canada had been traced to a fresh pressed apple beverage. These were the same fourteen children from the Toronto area that had spurred Karmali's work. The Hospital for Sick Children in Toronto normally sees five to ten patients with HUS per year, so to have fourteen in ten days was remarkable. Most of the children were from Pickering, a Toronto suburb twenty miles to the east. They had attended an outdoor fair where they drank apple juice. These children were very ill. One was comatose for three weeks; another was on a ventilator for several days. Six required dialysis and one infant died.

So it was clear that apple cider could make people sick.

The epidemiologists' next step was to determine precisely how the bacteria had got into the cider. From the clustering of cases (no new ones had been found for three weeks after the four girls first got sick), they surmised that only one or two batches of the cider had been contaminated. The Old Swanzey Orchard is a small local operation. The owner was very cooperative with the investigation (and the establishment no longer makes the cider).

Most of the apples used at Old Swanzey were drops—apples that had fallen off the trees naturally. The apples were neither brushed nor washed and were stored in open bins. The use of these unwashed dropped apples was forbidden by state regulation, although a later survey of cider producers found that both using drops for cider and not washing them first were fairly common practices. Cattle, the most common reservoir of *E. coli*, grazed in the same orchards where the drops were harvested. Deer, another animal that can carry the bacteria, were also common in these fields. The investigators cultured the cattle, the employees, the cider production equipment, and the water. They even visited deer tracking stations to culture freshly killed animals, all in an attempt to provide the decisive last link in the chain, but they never actually found the bacteria.

Nonetheless, both Drs. Lett and Besser agree that the most likely cause was deer, or possibly cattle, which had shed the bacteria on the ground where the dropped fruit had fallen. "It's well known that animals tend to shed the bacteria for short periods of time," says Dr. Besser.

Emily's condition gradually improved. On December 6, she was discharged. Fortunately, she never developed any neurological complications and did not require long-term dialysis. By December 10, her creatinine had fallen to 1.2. In fact, all four girls from Fall River recovered.

The doctors went on to prove that the *E. coli* could live in cider for much longer than anyone had previously thought. Further studies also showed that while one preservative (sodium benzoate) greatly shortened the time the bacteria survived in cider, another (potassium sorbate) actually prolonged it! The public health officials and the cider industry learned (or relearned) some valuable lessons about cider production, which will hopefully make cider even safer to drink than it already is. In their final report, the doctors recommended that consumers not drink cider made from apples that haven't been brushed and washed. The only way to know this may be to ask the proprietor of small cider operations.

The doctors' survey of the cider industry found that larger producers were far more likely to wash and brush their apples.

Since the Fall River outbreak, HUS and *E. coli* O157:H7 illnesses have become much more common, including some instances that affected many more victims. Other outbreaks have been small but interesting. In one, a local hospital in Rockford, Illinois, reported five cases of *E. coli* diarrhea. The common link was that the patients, all children, had been swimming in a lake in the area. Once investigators began looking, they found seven more cases. No adjacent cattle farms or sewage facilities were present, and the scientists considered the possibilities that waterfowl droppings or human excretion from a swimmer could have been the cause.

In three more recent outbreaks, children were infected at petting zoos in 2004–2005, in North Carolina (108 cases of *E. coli*, 15 with HUS), Florida (63 cases, 7 with HUS), and Arizona (2 cases). The children had been touching and feeding the animals or were exposed to animal manure from the wood shavings or sawdust in the pens.

Much larger multi-state outbreaks of *E. coli* O157:H7 have occurred. Widespread infections of this kind result from standard practices in the meatpacking industry, where small numbers of infected cattle can contaminate huge amounts of beef. Meat that does become contaminated may end up being distributed all across the country. In 1997, Hudson Foods recalled 25 million pounds of ground beef. In 2002, Pilgrim's Pride recalled more than 27 million pounds of poultry, and in 2006, the Topps Meat Company recalled over 21 million pounds of beef. This is only a partial list, and meat recalls are becoming increasingly common.

The CDC estimates that 3 to 7 percent of people infected with this strain of *E. coli* will develop HUS, of whom about 5 percent will die. And *E. coli* O157:H7 infects about 73,000 Americans annually. This translates into 2,168 hospitalizations and 61 deaths. These figures seem to be increasing over time.

Because cattle and other mammals often graze in fields that produce crops, such as lettuce and spinach, these foods have also been contaminated with *E. coli* and have resulted in large multi-state outbreaks. It is unlikely that we will ever eradicate the organism from our food supply.

And that is why food hygiene is so important. Washing fruits and vegetables can prevent the disease. Cooking hamburger so that the internal temperature is at least 155 degrees will kill the bacteria.

As for Emily, she is now a happy and healthy six-year-old. She is much more certain than the usual child her age when asked what she wants to be when she grows up—a doctor. "She plays with her doctor kit," says Peter, "and tells me I can be her nurse and work for her when she's the doctor."

And one other thing, she *never* drinks apple cider.

PART TWO   *The External Environment*

"When I first saw her, she was nontoxic looking, did not have a fever and was very interactive, but she couldn't speak properly; the words were slurred," recalls Dr. Fred Henretig, a pediatric emergency physician and toxicologist at Children's Hospital of Philadelphia (CHOP). His patient was Annie (as I'll call her), a five-year-old girl who had been transferred to the emergency department at CHOP for evaluation of a baffling and frightening constellation of symptoms. Little Annie had been a perfectly normal and healthy child until the day before her visit with Dr. Henretig in May 2003.

After day care that day, Annie began to squint because, she said, she couldn't see right. That evening, the brown-haired girl began to complain to her parents that she was seeing double and could see well only with one eye closed. She looked fine, however, and there were no obvious problems, so off to bed she went. But at 4 AM she woke up, crying that she couldn't see anything because she was seeing two of everything, and she was clenching her hands repeatedly. Her mother, a veterinarian, noticed that Annie's speech was slurred and she couldn't sit up or walk. Naturally, her mother was alarmed and rushed her daughter off to the emergency department at their local hospital.

The emergency physician working that shift at the hospital in Burlington County in southern New Jersey was equally alarmed. He was confronted with a little girl who had a highly abnormal neurological examination. His little patient was weak, could not speak properly, and had double vision. Her eyes could not move in tandem. In addition, she was ataxic, meaning she could not walk properly. This combination of symptoms—double vision and abnormal gait—suggests a problem with the back, or posterior, portion of the brain and demands a rapid and thorough evaluation.

Unlike chameleons, whose two eyes can move independently, humans are endowed with eyes that track objects only as a paired unit. Although there may be times when a human wishes for a lizard-like view of the environment, in fact the hard wiring in the brain that lets our eyes move together is dazzling. Three separate nerves control eye movements on each side. The nuclei that control each of these nerves lie in different parts of the brain; consequently, another set of electrical cables attach the three nuclei together. So the three nerves, three of the twelve cranial nerves, act in tight unison, yoked together. These cranial nerves (numbers three, four, and six of the twelve) in turn travel from the brain to the sets of ocular muscles that surround the eyes and control the direction that they move.

No matter how fast we move our heads, or how fast an object darts across our visual field, we see only one of it. We take this for granted. But when considering what is happening in the brain, the cranial nerves, and the ocular muscles, it is really quite remarkable. When we track an object moving from right to left, various electrical impulses race to the control centers and tell the eyes what to do. The left eye has to start out looking laterally while the right eye starts out looking medially, and then both eyes track toward the right as the object moves. One cranial nerve nucleus controls the lateral movement of the left eye, and a different one controls the medial movement of the right eye. As the object crosses the midline (our nose), this sequence reverses. If there is a vertical component to the movement, other nerves are involved.

Were it not for this yoking system, a catcher could not catch a pitched ball and each pass in basketball would be an accident waiting to happen. When this system collapses, we see two of everything.

Double vision—or diplopia, as the doctors call it—is a very disconcerting symptom to patients; it's not the way we're used to seeing the world and it is frightening when it happens. For doctors too, this symptom is a worrisome one, because the list of conditions that cause diplopia is relatively short, and for the most part consists of serious medical conditions.

A problem anywhere along the neurological pathway can result in double vision. A stroke or a multiple sclerosis plaque placed near the nucleus of the command centers can lead to double vision. Any problem that hits the nerve along its course to the ocular muscles can have the same effect. Potential problems include tumors, an aneurysm in the arteries around the brain that physically compress the nerve, and inflammation of the nerves. Because each one of these is such a serious problem, double vision is a symptom that demands a rapid and thorough evaluation.

So the physician at the local hospital initiated a workup that included a wide array of blood and urine tests. The basic blood work—red and white blood cell counts, routine chemistries like blood sugar and sodium—all came back normal. As one might predict from the list of potential causes of double vision, these basic tests did not result in any diagnosis.

So the emergency physician next ordered sophisticated brain scans, including an MRI (magnetic resonance imaging) and an MRA (magnetic resonance angiography). When the radiologist looked at the MRI, he thought there was diminished flow to one of the arteries at the back of the brain. Translation: Annie might be having a stroke, an odd problem for a five-year-old.

Stroke is a common problem in adults; in fact, it is the third leading cause of death and the leading cause of disability. But it's distinctly uncommon in children. So the emergency physician did what any prudent doctor would do; he transferred his patient to a tertiary care facility, in this case CHOP, where world-class experts in pediatric neurology could lend their expertise to the case.

And this is where our story opened, sometime in the late afternoon as Annie was ushered into the emergency department at CHOP with an armful of diagnostic studies and a diagnosis of "presumed stroke." Dr. Henretig's observation that his little patient looked well is an important one. How sick or well a patient looks to a doctor often dictates the pace that an evaluation will take place, whether that patient is admitted or discharged, and whether medications are started or not, and if they are, whether it is by mouth or intravenously. But although first impressions are important, Dr. Henretig was well aware that despite the fact that she looked well, Annie's neurological condition was precarious, and determining the cause for her symptoms was the first step toward fixing it. So he was reassured by her overall appearance, but Dr. Henretig took careful stock of the puzzling array of signs and symptoms that he was confronted with.

As is common in emergency medicine, Dr. Henretig started pursuing multiple tasks simultaneously. He wanted his own radiology staff to review the films done at the outside hospital. And he ordered a consultation with neurologists to get their input. But while arranging for these things to be accomplished, he carefully examined Annie.

Her vital signs were essentially normal, with the exception of a slightly rapid pulse rate. But there was no fever, no problems with her ability to breathe and get oxygen into her blood. Her blood pressure was normal. The specialist pediatric neuroradiologists reviewed the MR scans from the original hospital and thought that they were normal. The diagnosis of stroke became much less likely.

But there were obvious and disturbing abnormalities in her neurological function. Her eye movements (the sixth cranial nerve in this particular case) were clearly abnormal; neither eye could look outward from the midline. This finding accounted for her double vision. And Annie's face was twisted to one side due to facial paralysis. This is known commonly as a Bell's, or facial nerve, palsy, an indication that her seventh cranial nerve was also not working properly. The difficulty in walking that the doctor in the first emergency department had noticed was because she was so profoundly weak. Not only could she not walk properly, she could barely sit up by herself. Dr. Henretig's leading diagnosis was Guillain-Barré syndrome.

Guillain-Barré syndrome is a condition whereby the peripheral nerve roots, as they exit from the spinal cord, cease to function normally. It is an unusual problem; the nerve roots are thought to become inflamed following some other trouble in the body, such as a trivial upper respiratory infection, a bout of gastroenteritis, or sometimes an immunization.

Guillain-Barré syndrome was first reported in 1859 by a French physician, Jean-Baptiste-Octave Landry de Thézillat. He reported ten cases, half of whom he personally attended. Of those five, two died from respiratory failure. One of the fatal cases was a thirty-four-year-old paver who, on June 1, 1859, walked into the hospital complaining of some weakness and funny sensations in his feet. By the third week his limbs were paralyzed, and he developed difficulty breathing, chewing, and swallowing. Shortly thereafter, he died. The disease became known as ascending paralysis of Landry, and his original description remains accurate to this day.

He wrote: "The main problem is usually a motor disorder characterized by a gradual diminution of muscular strength and flaccid limbs and without contractures, convulsions or reflex movements of any kind. In almost all cases, micturition and defecation remain normal. One does not observe any symptoms referable to the central nervous system. . . . The intellectual faculties are preserved until the end. The onset of paralysis can be preceded by a general feeling of weakness, pins and needles, and even slight cramps. . . . The weakness spreads rapidly from the lower to the upper parts of the body with a universal tendency to become generalized. . . . When the paralysis reaches its maximum intensity the danger of asphyxia is always imminent. However in eight out of ten cases, death was avoided, either by skillful professional intervention or a spontaneous remission of this phase of the illness."

Decades later, in 1916, three other French physicians (George Guillain, Jean-Alexandre Barré, and André Strohl) described two more cases of what seemed to be the same problem. Guillain and Barré were medical students together who ended up as military doctors. They described two soldiers who became paralyzed for no apparent reason. The patients' symptoms were similar to those described by Landry—muscle weakness, loss of reflexes, and a gradual progression from the lower extremities to the upper—but both of them recovered. When the doctors did a spinal tap (which had not yet been developed when Landry was practicing), they found an elevated protein level but no white blood cells in the spinal fluid. The absence of cells was important, since two conditions that were common at the time and that could cause similar symptoms, tuberculosis and syphilis, were associated with cells in the spinal fluid.

Over the following years, they described additional cases. Although some coined the moniker Landry-Guillain-Barré syndrome, Guillain was angered by the addition of Landry's name and argued that Landry's cases were not really the same condition, in part because their spinal fluid was not tested and in part because some of Landry's patients died. Over time, Landry's name was dropped. And somehow the name of Strohl, who never really got much billing, suffered the same fate. So today, doctors commonly refer to this form of ascending paralysis as Guillain-Barré syndrome.

The syndrome often follows an acute infection, often of the gastrointestinal or upper respiratory tract, and sometimes it follows a vaccination. In the 1970s, Guillain-Barré flashed into the headlines after an excess in cases was found in the wake of the swine-flu immunization campaign. Patients experience weakness, usually starting with the lower extremities and then ascending to the arms and to the respiratory muscles, including the diaphragm. When the diaphragm stops working, the patient can no longer breathe, and without prompt intervention will die.

Before the advent of modern intensive care units, approximately 20–30 percent of patients with Guillain-Barré died. In a ten-year review of cases from Ethiopia published in 2005, investigators found a mortality rate of 26 percent, a dismal statistic that they ascribed to poor access to intensive care in that country. In developed countries, the mortality rate is closer to 2–4 percent, because with modern ICU-level supportive care, patients can be kept alive on a breathing machine until the nerve damage improves. Today, treatment of Guillain-Barré is by plasma exchange or intravenous immunoglobulin. Neither is a benign therapy. Before treatment can be initiated, however, the correct diagnosis must be established. Other diseases can mimic Guillain-Barré syndrome, and these other problems have completely different treatments.

Weakness, for example, could be from a tumor, blood clot, or abscess that is compressing the spinal cord. The treatments for these problems might involve surgery to remove a clot or tumor, or powerful antibiotics to treat an infection. Other times, the spinal cord itself might be inflamed. This could be from diseases as diverse as multiple sclerosis, Lyme disease, or even schistosomiasis, caused by a parasite from the Nile that can affect the spine.

But five-year-old Annie had not been to any such exotic locations. So Dr. Henretig's leading diagnosis was a type of Guillain-Barré syndrome called the Miller-Fisher variant, named for a Canadian neurologist, Charles Miller Fisher, who first described it in 1956. In this syndrome, there is prominent involvement with the cranial nerves. The diagnostic test that Dr. Henretig wanted to perform was a spinal tap, or lumbar puncture. In this procedure, after cleaning the skin of the back with a potent antiseptic solution and numbing the area with a local anesthetic, the physician places a needle into the space between two adjacent bones of the spine. The needle pierces the outer covering of the spinal cord to the area where the spinal fluid lies. The exact location of the needle is a couple of inches lower than the bottom end of the actual spinal cord. Through the needle, he draws out a small quantity of cerebrospinal fluid, which acts as a shock absorber and nutrient source for the brain and spinal cord. This fluid is normally crystal clear and looks like water. The pressure is measured, and the fluid is sent to the hospital laboratory to be tested for protein levels and cell counts. The microbiology lab will determine if there is an infection. The major clue to the diagnosis of Guillain-Barré syndrome is the dual findings of elevated protein level with a normal cell count, as described back in 1916.

To do this procedure in children, physicians will sometimes administer a combination of medications through an intravenous line, to ease the pain and allay the anxiety and fear that a patient will feel when having a spinal tap. This is called intravenous procedural sedation. Dr. Henretig's associate Dr. Jill Posner and her staff sedated Annie and performed the spinal tap. As it usually does, the procedure went smoothly, and the fluid was sent off to the lab.

One of the other pediatric emergency specialists who was taking care of Annie was Dr. Reza Daugherty. He remembers: "We talked to the neurologists. They came down in a team with like six people: the attending, the fellow, a resident, and some medical students. Annie was areflexic at that point. Because she had lost her reflexes, and given the clinical scenario, we all thought that the Miller-Fisher variant of Guillain-Barré was the most likely diagnosis." Annie was starting to have respiratory problems by this point. The doctors tested her lung function by measuring what is called a negative inspiratory force, to see how well the respiratory muscles are working. Annie's showed some signs of deterioration.

"She was going to go to pediatric ICU to get plasmapheresis," recalls Daugherty, "and she was likely going to need to be put on a ventilator. The mother started getting nervous when they talked about the large lines necessary for the plasmapheresis." The treatment of plasmapheresis involves placing a large intravenous line into a central vein of the body. There are potential complications, both from inserting the large line and from the treatment itself. Plasmapheresis is in some ways similar to hemodialysis, used for patients with kidney failure. Several treatments are done over a week or ten days, during which large volumes of blood plasma are drawn off into a machine, where various proteins and antibodies are removed before the plasma is returned to the patient. The precise mechanism of how this treatment works is unknown, but it clearly improves the outcomes for many patients.

The results of Annie's spinal fluid analysis returned: there were no cells, but the protein level was also normal. However, the normal findings did not definitively exclude a diagnosis of Guillain-Barré; in fact, many times early in the progression, the spinal fluid is normal, and Annie had been sick for less than twenty-four hours.

Dr. Posner recalls: "Even with the procedural sedation, she was very fretful and unhappy during the spinal tap. Afterward, she was rolled up in her mom's lap. And her mother started to caress her hair to comfort her. At some point, the mother thought she felt something abnormal just behind one ear, and parted her hair." The "something," Annie's mother quickly realized, was a fully engorged tick. She called to the nurse and doctor. Since the mother was a veterinarian, she removed the tick.

The significance of the tick cannot be overstated, and it threw a curve ball into the whole analysis. Lyme disease is an extremely common affliction in southern New Jersey. And Lyme disease can sometimes cause transverse myelitis—an inflammation of the spinal cord that can be confused with Guillain-Barré syndrome. Lyme disease can also cause the cranial nerve problems that Annie had. And the time of year was also right. Late spring and early summer are the peak season for Lyme disease. However, neurological symptoms from Lyme disease follow the tick bite by weeks to months, and are never found while the tick is still attached. Finally, this tick wasn't right for that. Lyme disease is caused by bacteria spread by the bite of an infected *Ixodes* tick, usually referred to as the deer tick. These ticks are very small, even when fully engorged. The tick that was removed from Annie's scalp was not a deer tick; it was a *Dermacentor*, or common dog tick—not the kind that causes Lyme at all.

These much larger ticks are the vectors of all sorts of infectious agents. They carry the bacteria that cause Rocky Mountain spotted fever and tularemia and ehrlichiosis. They carry some viruses as well. But there is one disease that *Dermacentor* ticks cause that is not an infection at all: tick paralysis. This results not from a bacteria or virus passed along by ticks but from a neurotoxin that the ticks themselves produce in their salivary glands. However, tick paralysis is an extraordinarily rare disease, and it is virtually nonexistent in New Jersey. The vast majority of doctors go through their entire professional careers without ever seeing a single case of tick paralysis. Even at CHOP, with the collective experience of the emergency physicians and the neurologists, none had ever seen a case. Finding this tick changed everything though, and Annie's doctors were cautiously optimistic.

"At that point," says Posner, "we figured that tick paralysis was the correct diagnosis, and if we were right, we had already treated it [by removing the tick]. But because none of us had ever seen a case, we still admitted her to the ICU because we didn't know what to expect."

Tick paralysis is a disease of both humans and animals that occurs worldwide. In North America, it is most commonly seen in the western United States and Canada, but even in these areas it is quite rare. In one series of cases from the state of Washington, only thirty-three instances were identified over a fifty-year period. Tick paralysis mimics Guillain-Barré syndrome; it presents as an ascending bilateral flaccid paralysis, although it usually progresses over hours to days, faster than the typical case of Guillain-Barré. The neurotoxin is produced when the female ticks of certain species feed. A tick that remains attached to a human or animal, feeding on its blood, secretes the toxin into the host's bloodstream. Over the course of several days, the toxin is absorbed, and paralysis rapidly ensues. Also like Guillain-Barré, sensory function is spared, but as the paralysis tightens its grip on the victim, the respiratory muscles fail, and without intervention, many patients die.

Once diagnosed, the treatment is simplicity itself—remove the tick. Within hours, patients begin to show meaningful signs of improvement. This is because, unlike with Lyme disease or other tick-borne infections, it's not an infection at all that is causing the symptoms. Once the tick is removed, it stops secreting the toxin into the victim, and the toxin is cleared from the body and the nerves begin to work normally again. But if the tick is not found, some patients, as much as 12 percent, will die from the condition. Patients whose diagnoses remain obscure may stop breathing and require a ventilator to survive.

In others, the offending tick probably feeds to repletion and then falls off, and the patient improves, possibly without ever being correctly diagnosed. As with any extremely rare disease, many patients with tick paralysis are not properly diagnosed, at least not initially, because the condition mimics more common problems.

The earliest reference to tick paralysis in humans dates back to 1824, in Australia. In that year, William Howell referred in his diary to a certain tick, "which buries itself in the flesh and would in the end destroy either man or beast if not removed in time." The first two reports of tick paralysis in North America appeared independently in 1912. One resulted from inquiries to physicians in British Columbia to learn whether Rocky Mountain spotted fever was present in their province. The responses from the physicians suggested nine cases of tick paralysis. That same year, an Oregon physician summarized reports of twelve cases that had occurred in Oregon and Idaho, three of which were fatal.

A year later, a young pathologist named Seymour Hadwen was sent by the Department of Agriculture of British Columbia to investigate an outbreak of paralysis in sheep. One farmer had reported that, each spring for the previous three years, his sheep had been dying from paralysis. The local veterinarians had looked into the matter but were stumped. When Hadwen started his investigation, he found a fully engorged tick on the back of one recently paralyzed lamb. Two months later, he observed that, in another lamb, which was paralyzed in the hindquarters only, removal of an engorged tick was associated with rapid improvement in the animal's condition. Wise enough to discuss the situation with local farmers, Hadwen learned that other animals—horses, birds, rabbits, and dogs—also became paralyzed in the same way.

Hadwen was aware of what little information existed at this time in the medical literature and began to investigate further. He experimented with three lambs, allowing ticks to feed on them, and found that as the female ticks engorged, usually after six to eight days of feeding, he could reproduce the paralysis. He also observed that when he removed the ticks, the animals recovered. From these and other experiments, he made three deductions. First, the symptoms were clearly related to the feeding of adult female *Dermacentor* ticks and would begin to occur at about day six. Second, he theorized that the illness starts when the tick injects a toxin coincident in time with when the tick has completely engorged. He thought an infectious agent was unlikely. Last, he observed that the progression of symptoms from isolated hindquarter weakness to total paralysis, including respiratory failure, was rapid and predictable. He added, "It would appear advisable . . . to remove the ticks from the affected animals."

Hadwen's observations remain accurate nearly a century later. In humans, there is a tendency for tick paralysis to occur in children, probably because, pound for pound, the dose of the toxin in children is higher than in adults. Among children, girls are affected more often than boys; the likely explanation is that many young girls have long hair, which makes it harder to see the ticks, allowing them to feed undetected long enough to secrete their toxin. The ticks that produce tick paralysis can feed for a week or more, and it usually takes one that has been feeding for about five days to cause symptoms.

Because tick paralysis is so rare, it's frequently misdiagnosed, often as Guillain-Barré syndrome. In one series of six patients from Mississippi, all were initially diagnosed with Guillain-Barré; in one five-year-old girl, the correct diagnosis was made only after she was already receiving treatment for that problem. While the mother was bathing the child in the ICU, she found an engorged tick and removed it. The child rapidly improved. The same thing happened when a nurse in Colorado found an engorged tick on the scalp of a six-year-old while she bathed her. This youngster was on a ventilator in the ICU for presumed Guillain-Barré syndrome.

There is a long list of other instances in which the diagnosis was made almost by accident. One was a six-year-old girl from Georgia, on whom a pediatric doctor in training found a tick while he was preparing to insert a central intravenous catheter for plasmapheresis. In that case, three pediatricians, a pediatric neurologist, and an intensive care specialist had all missed the tick. In another, while a technician was applying electrodes for an electroencephalogram (EEG) onto the scalp of a three-year-old, the child's mother found a tick. In a case from North Carolina, an MRI scan showed a tick embedded in the scalp. So it is completely understandable that the diagnosis could be missed initially.

"She was down in the emergency department for a while," Dr. Posner recalls about Annie, "and before she went upstairs to the ICU, I remember her saying, 'I don't see double anymore, Mom!' By the next morning, her symptoms had improved 99 percent, and twelve hours after that, she was entirely normal." Annie recovered fully, and the next day she was discharged from the hospital feeling perfectly well. This was a happy ending for Annie, but as it turned out, it was not the end of the story.

On July 22, two months to the day after Annie's presentation, Dr. Reza Daugherty got a phone call. "We do the medical command for transports of patients that are being referred to CHOP from outside hospitals. I was in the office that day, and carrying the medical command pager, when I got a call from an outside hospital. The doctor on the line said, 'We've got this little girl with ataxia and weakness . . .' the story began." The doctor from the referring facility relayed a familiar tale. He had a seven-year-old who began complaining of pain in both legs and then, over the next twenty-four hours, became so weak that she could not walk. As a result of her weakness and clumsiness, she could not feed herself because she could not bring a fork to her mouth.

"At the outside hospital," recalls Daugherty, "they did some routine blood work and a brain CT scan; all the results were normal. They diagnosed Guillain-Barré syndrome. I asked that they not do any further tests or the lumbar puncture, but to just transfer the patient to us. I remember saying to the transport nurse, 'this sounds like that last case but there's no way she's got tick paralysis.' It was early afternoon when she physically got to the emergency department. I was in the office, but I ran down to see her as soon as she arrived. I remember that the mom was remarkably calm. The resident was already examining the girl. She was moderately weak in the lower extremities and slightly so in her arms. Her right eyelid was a bit droopy, and she was very clumsy when moving her arms and legs.

"By now, she was about twelve hours into her course. She had very long straight hair. When I examined her scalp, to my amazement, I found an engorged tick in almost the exact same location as in the first patient. I explained the situation to the parents, who were beginning to get anxious, and I removed the tick. By thinking of the diagnosis [and then finding the tick and removing it], we avoided all the imaging tests, the spinal tap, and the ICU admission. She began feeling better within two to three hours, and in eighteen hours, she felt normal and went home.

With two cases of a rare and potentially fatal disease presenting to the same hospital in such a brief period of time, the physicians at CHOP notified the CDC in Atlanta. The CDC posted a notice on its Internet epidemic information exchange site on July 29, 2003. Following protocol, the epidemiologists also notified the New Jersey Department of Health and Senior Services. The state officials were fairly sure that the two cases represented just a very unusual coincidence. Nevertheless, they held a press conference to notify and warn the public. The commissioner of the department, Clifton Lacey, said: "Tick paralysis is very rare in this part of the country. This is extremely interesting to us. This may be the first two cases in New Jersey. Clearly we have not heard of cases in at least three decades."

He and his staff got the word out to parents about the importance of regular tick checks on their children. There were newspaper articles and television interviews. After receiving permission from the two families involved, the department conducted further interviews of those involved and evaluated their risk factors. These investigations did not find anything out of the ordinary for a dog-owning suburban family in southern New Jersey. In the end, the state officials were correct: it appeared to be a very unusual coincidence; no further cases were diagnosed.

Dr. Daugherty recalls: "It was really amazing when I saw the second case; I was shocked that it could be true—to see two cases of such a rare disease in so short a period of time. I also felt terrific at how easy it was to ease the parents' anxiety. I told them that I had seen a little girl with the same thing two months before and that she did very well. The ironic thing about the first case was that after about twenty doctors had seen the patient, and having lots of tests including an MRI and a spinal tap, that it was the mom who really made the diagnosis."

~~~~~~~

"I got sick the first time in December," recalls Philip Bradford (as I'll call him). "At first I thought it was just the flu—the usual cough, fevers, chest pain, just feeling lousy, but it lasted a few weeks. When it didn't clear up, I saw my doctor, who prescribed first erythromycin and then a tetracycline-type drug. Finally, he ordered a chest x-ray, which showed pneumonia. A month later, there was still no improvement, so he hospitalized me and I had a whole array of tests."

These included skin tests for tuberculosis, sputum cultures for more conventional bacteria, a biopsy of a suspicious lymph node from the area just above Bradford's collarbone, and a bronchoscopy—a test in which a rigid scope is inserted through the throat and into the large bronchial tubes so that the physician can directly inspect the air passages in the lungs. This was in 1973, before CT scans of the chest, so he also had special lung x-rays called tomograms, where conventional x-ray machines narrowed their field of focus to examine thin slices of the lung in greater detail. The tomograms showed clusters of nodules in both lungs that were very concerning to the doctor. Despite this extensive evaluation, however, the physician was unable to make a definitive diagnosis, but he did reach a tentative one.

Remembers Bradford: "The doctor's conclusion, which he communicated to my wife in the hall outside of my room, was that I had lung cancer, and he advised a major operation to biopsy the lung. I will never forget that diagnosis."

The doctor thought the cancer had spread to the lungs from another, as yet undiscovered site. In order to make a definitive tissue diagnosis of this presumed metastatic cancer, he advised a thoracotomy—a major surgical procedure that is designed to open up the chest like a clamshell, so that suspicious tissues can be biopsied and examined under the microscope.

But Bradford, thirty-three years old, was not frightened. "I simply didn't believe that's what I had," he explains. "I was healthy and a non-smoker. I wanted a second opinion. My wife telephoned some physician relatives who ultimately put us in touch with Dr. Earl Wilkins. Dr. Wilkins spent a lot of time with me. He asked me a lot of questions and examined me from head to toe. He didn't know what I had, but he told me he didn't think it was cancer."

Dr. Earl W. Wilkins Jr., now retired but then a senior thoracic surgeon at the Massachusetts General Hospital in Boston, remembers the case clearly. "He brought a stack of records with him. I reviewed the medical records of the first hospitalization, then took my own history and carefully examined him," he recalls. "[Cancer] was what he and I were worried about when we first met. The tomograms obtained at the outside hospital demonstrated multiple nodular densities, four on the right side and two on the left, that were highly suggestive of metastatic cancer.

"[But] I was struck by two things: First, if this was metastatic cancer to the lung, I could detect no primary site. And second, I had the benefit of a longer time interval. Although the radiologist wasn't sure, I thought that one of the nodules on the latest x-ray was slightly smaller than it had been on a previous film. If that was true, a cancer would be very unlikely. Neither I nor the patient was inclined to go ahead with the thoracotomy."

Another factor that was in the back of Wilkins' mind was that if this was metastatic cancer that had already spread so extensively, there was little risk in waiting a short period of time. As it turned out, not doing the surgery was the right choice, because over the next few weeks, Bradford's symptoms, along with the nodules on the chest x-ray, vanished as mysteriously as they had appeared.

"I just gradually got better," recalls Bradford, an executive with a large banking firm. He worked in downtown Boston and lived in a small town on Boston's South Shore, in a marshy area, across from a farm. Despite the fact that there were no overt changes in his life, he remained well for almost a year. But then, in September 1974, he again started coughing and running a fever. And once again, his chest x-ray blossomed with ominous nodules; then, as with the previous episode, after a few weeks his symptoms mysteriously vanished.

This time, Wilkins sent him to see Dr. Robert H. Rubin, an infectious disease specialist at Mass General, and now director of the hospital's clinical investigation program. "At the time I was doing some general internal medicine as well as infectious diseases. After reviewing [all of the records from the first hospitalization], I was immediately impressed by three aspects of the case," Rubin recalls. "First was that Bradford appeared healthy and athletic, not the picture of someone with a chronic disease. Second, between episodes, he continued to jog over five miles with no apparent problem. And third, his physical examination was normal."

Rubin reasoned that if the nodules that appeared on the x-rays were always in the same location, then a chronic structural or anatomical lesion within the lung would be the likeliest cause. However, each x-ray showed that different parts of the lungs were involved during different episodes. The first time it was the right middle lobe and both lower lobes; the next time, it was the upper lobes. "There were clearly different segments of the lung involved each time. Therefore," says Rubin, "it must have been something in the environment. And because none of the multiple tests had revealed the presence of a microbe that might have been the culprit, the question of hypersensitivity pneumonia immediately arose."

Pneumonia, or more properly, pneumonitis, simply means inflammation of the lung. The cause of that inflammation could be anything—bacteria, a virus, a chemical, or even radiation. In typical infectious pneumonia, the bacteria or virus directly causes damage to tissue. In an attempt to kill the invading pathogen, the body mounts a cellular and chemical war. The body's immune system—antibodies and various types of specialized white blood cells called lymphocytes, plasma cells, and polymorphonuclear leukocytes—tries to contain the foreign material, and then kill it. Inflammation is the result of the clutter and debris left behind on the battlefield.

Hypersensitivity pneumonia occurs when a lung becomes inflamed in response to breathing air that contains organic dusts laden with biologic stowaways. These stowaways are typically small amounts of mold, or fungi or bacteria or spores that are drawn in by the normal flow of air and are small enough to be deposited deep into the lungs. They land in the alveoli, the functional units of the lung. Blood flows past these tiny air-filled sacs to facilitate the exchange of gases—oxygen in, carbon dioxide out—which is the lung's primary job. Although these biological stowaways are not necessarily as toxic or invasive as other viruses and bacteria that cause typical infectious pneumonia, the immune system still perceives them as foreign invaders and therefore seeks to contain them.

Just as with the more conventional pathogenic bacteria, this containment process causes inflammation. To the lung, inflammation is inflammation, regardless of the primary inciting event. Patients with hypersensitivity pneumonia develop nonspecific symptoms often within hours of being exposed to these dusts. And these symptoms, such as fever, chills, headache, cough, and shortness of breath, can be easily misdiagnosed as flu, bronchitis, or another kind of pneumonia, or in rare circumstances, a lung cancer.

That is, unless the doctor first thinks of the diagnosis and then asks some very specific questions. Generally, a patient with hypersensitivity pneumonia has been exposed to organic dust as a result of his or her job or hobby. The prototypical form is farmer's lung, a condition that develops when farmers working with hay inhale large amounts of spores from a group of bacteria called thermophilic actinomycetes.

The term itself is a mouthful, but anyone who has done any composting in the garden knows that these actinomycetes are really a noseful. They are an important element in composted soil, producing its characteristic earthy smell. The name actinomycete suggests a branching fungus, and in fact that's what scientists thought they were for many years. But in reality, they belong to the realm of bacteria that branch into long filaments and that resemble fungi in appearance. "Thermophilic" means heat loving. These organisms are most active at 120–150 degrees Fahrenheit.

Although physicians had recognized for centuries an association between exposure to dusts from farms and respiratory problems, the first and certainly one of the most colorful accounts of farmer's lung was published in the *British Medical Journal* by Dr. J. Munro Campbell, a tuberculosis officer in Grange-over-Sands, England, located in Westmorland County. He wrote:

> *The summer of 1931 proved a very bad season for hay-making in Westmorland, owing to rain, and much of the hay was eventually taken in in an unsatisfactorily damp condition. The inevitable result was the development of a great deal of mould, especially in the lower strata, so that working with it later produced dense clouds of "white" or "hay" dust, stated by those afflicted to be the worst they had ever experienced. In the ordinary course of farm-work, transient cough and wheeziness are recognized effects of contact with "white" dust, but in five of the cases which I had the opportunity of examining, the symptoms were so severe that they seem worth recording. These cases were seen during the period April to June, 1932, which in itself is significant as being the period when the supply of last year's hay was nearing the end.*
>
> *All the patients were farmers or farm labourers, whose ages ranged from 21 to 46 years, and whose previous health records were good. . . . The onset of [symptoms] was very similar in each case: a noticeable shortness of breath for some weeks previously whilst carrying out the normal routine, including work with hay, until a climax was reached by some specific act (for example, clearing out the remainder of the hay from a barn) and within 36 hours, the man was extremely [short of breath], a step or two being impossible, distressed, and cyanotic, and appeared almost in extremis.*
>
> *It was about three weeks later that most of these cases were seen by me, when doubts arose as to the possible existence of tuberculosis infection. . . . Later, when the patients were able to attend for x-ray examination, films showed a generalized, very fine granular stippling (reminiscent of, though much finer than, silicosis). . . . Several of these patients have been examined three to four months afterwards, and except [for one of them], have very gradually lost their shortness of breath. No other symptoms remained troublesome, and the chest signs later were practically negative. X-ray films now showed very little stippling.*
>
> *This "hay" dust, when allowed to settle on a clean plate, was found to be a soft, slaty-grey powder. Samples of the sputa were examined when ob-*

tainable, and showed no tubercle bacilli; though in one case a definite fungus was found, this finding was not repeated, either in this patient's or in any other patient's sputum and no other clues to a possible cause were found in the sputa. Though samples of the hay dust were examined and several fungi recognized, no evidence of any correlating factor could be found.

The "fungi" that Dr. Campbell saw were very likely thermophilic actinomycetes, which have been only recently reclassified as bacteria. Why would these bacteria be in a stack of hay in the first place? Nature always has a purpose, and aside from causing disease in these farmers, what possible grander purpose could these odiferous organisms serve? The answer to this question can be summarized in two words—decay and putrefaction.

Decay and putrefaction are as much a part of the natural cycle of life on this planet as birth and growth. In fact, the study of these natural destructive processes occupied much of the early work of no less than Louis Pasteur. Economic needs often propel scientific work, and Pasteur had been enlisted to help the French beer industry, which was being decimated by decay and putrefaction. In a presentation that he delivered in 1863, titled "Investigation into the Role Attributed to Atmospheric Oxygen Gas in the Destruction of Animal and Vegetable Substances After Death," he said:

> *Fermentation, putrefaction, and slow combustion are the three phenomena which concur in the accomplishment of this great fact of the destruction of organic substances—a condition necessary for the maintenance of life on the earth. . . .*
>
> *. . . In every case, life, manifesting itself in the lowest forms of organization, appears to me to be one of the essential conditions of these phenomena, but life of a nature unknown hitherto; that is to say, without consumption of air or of free oxygen.*
>
> . . . This leads to the general conclusion that life controls the work of death in all its phases, and that the three terms of that perpetual return to the atmosphere, and to the mineral kingdom, of the elements which vegetables and animals have abstracted from

them, are correlative acts of development and of the multiplication of organized beings. . . . *[emphasis added]*

> *But [it] is worthy of remark and this is precisely the principal fact to which I today wish to draw the attention of the Academy: the slow combustion of organic substances after death, however real, is barely perceptible when the air is deprived of the germs of lower organisms. It becomes rapid, considerable, not to be compared with the former situation, should the organic substances be covered by moulds . . .*

Translation: living organisms are necessary for the process of decay. This was a radical departure from the status quo, and the significance of Pasteur's discovery cannot be overstated. His experiments showed for the first time that the decay of organisms was in fact a biological and not a purely chemical process. The findings from this same series of experiments partly led to his attack on contemporary scientists who believed in the spontaneous generation of life.

Since Pasteur's time, scientists have learned that one of the most important agents of biological decay is the group of bacteria called the thermophilic actinomycetes, which are the primary decomposers of tough plant materials like bark, leaves, and stems. In the warm environment of a compost heap, they are especially effective at attacking the components of raw plant tissues, such as cellulose, chitin, and lignin. Other types of microorganisms and insects complete the decay cycle, converting organic matter back into inorganic substances. These inorganic substances become the building blocks for the next generation of living organisms. This process is important not just for creating fertilizer. Imagine the result if the fallen leaves from tens of thousands of years of trees never decomposed. The entire earth would be buried beneath them. As Pasteur recognized, the job thermophilic actinomycetes do is essential to life itself.

Unfortunately, however, the spores from these necessary actinomycetes happen to be a perfect size for being inhaled into the lungs of humans. It has been estimated that farmers working in an area where moldy hay is disturbed could inhale approximately 750,000 actinomycete spores per minute.

Farmers are not the only ones at risk, either. The same syndrome occurs in pigeon breeders and parakeet fanciers. People who harvest sugarcane and coffee beans, or those who cure tobacco, or anyone who works with wood dust, cheese, maple bark, mushrooms, soybean feed, and barley can get hypersensitivity pneumonia. Cases have been ascribed to exposure to moldy shower curtains and moist saxophone mouthpieces. The list continues to grow. In the absence of an obvious source of exposure, in which case the patient will often have already made the connection, a doctor needs to take a meticulously detailed occupational and environmental history to make an accurate diagnosis.

Philip Bradford, however, was not a farmer, or a pigeon breeder or a harvester of sugarcane, or anything else on that expansive list of potential causes. He was a banker.

If Rubin's suspicion was true, then there was a missing piece of information, and he was determined to find it. "When I was a senior resident at the Peter Bent Brigham Hospital, Professor J. Pepys from the Brompton Hospital in London was a visiting professor," says Rubin, "and I was 'in charge' of him for the week. He did some of the pioneering work in hypersensitivity pneumonia, and he had written a book on allergic diseases of the lung." Rubin had read that book, and he knew that the devil (or in this case, the diagnosis) was in the details.

As described in the written report of the case in the *New England Journal of Medicine*, Rubin uncovered the following potential exposures that Bradford had encountered. "Thirteen years earlier he had joined the Air Force, and during the next four years, he was stationed in Vietnam, Texas, central United States and Europe. Subsequently, he resided in New England and traveled only to Detroit and Chicago. For approximately a year and a half before admission [to the hospital], he worked in a new high-rise building in Boston. A pet dog had been recently examined by a veterinarian and reported to be normal. There was no history of allergy except for mild seasonal hay fever that began at the age of 20 years."

Although Bradford's job did not put him at risk for a textbook case of hypersensitivity pneumonia, Rubin knew that modern times bring modern risks. Investigators have reported people who have developed hypersensitivity pneumonia because of organisms circulated by air conditioners and humidifiers. "I questioned Bradford at length about humidifiers, his home heating system, hobbies, but I couldn't come up with any exposures that would account for his symptoms," Rubin explained.

Bradford recalls that Rubin took "an exhaustive personal history. I had spent a year in Vietnam in the air force, and there was some speculation that I had some exotic something-or-other that I had brought back from Southeast Asia."

Finally, from the extensive lists of questions and the meticulous lines of inquiry, one clue emerged. The symptoms had begun shortly after Bradford's firm moved into a new office space. The new building was similar in design to so many modern structures that punctuated the Boston skyline in the 1970s—essentially a concrete box studded with smoked-glass windows. Like most workers in modern high-rises, Bradford was entirely at the mercy of a heating, ventilation, and air-conditioning (HVAC) system for his air supply. Such buildings are effectively sealed off from the fresh air outside, and Rubin thought his patient could be reacting to something that the HVAC system had exposed him to.

But that theory had at least two glaring problems. "He went into the office every day. Why would the symptoms be intermittent? And if it was the office, why weren't other co-workers getting sick?" Rubin wondered. Then he thought of a possible solution to the first of these difficulties with the theory.

"It became apparent that the new building was fraught with problems involving the ductwork. I asked Mr. Bradford to get copies of the maintenance records of the HVAC duct from the building managers to find out exactly when the air had been blown back and forth and when repair work had been done on the ductwork going into his office," explained Rubin. "When he brought them back to me, sure enough, they revealed a possible explanation. The system was cleaned by forcing air through the ducts under pressure. The duct system had been blown clean twice. And it jived perfectly with the timing of the patient's symptoms. Within the first day after major ductwork had been done during working hours, he experienced an episode of pulmonary infiltrates [nodules on the chest x-ray]."

Rubin's next step was to send a sample of Bradford's blood to the Harvard School of Public Health for analysis. He ordered a precipitin test, which Dr. Pepys had helped to develop. In this test, the patient's blood is mixed with a preparation of thermophilic actinomycetes to see if antibodies in the blood will clump—or precipitate—with an antigen from the bacteria.

Although the owners of the building thought Rubin's hypothesis was somewhat farfetched, there were precedents. Four years earlier, Dr. Edward Banaszak and his colleagues reported a cluster of hypersensitivity pneumonia cases in the *New England Journal of Medicine.* Their report described the travails of four office workers who had developed fever, chills, cough, and shortness of breath. They demonstrated that the air-conditioning system in the office where the victims worked harbored thermophilic actinomycetes. The patients all had a positive precipitin test. After a thorough cleaning and modification of the system, all four patients were cured.

Then the results of Bradford's blood test returned—negative.

Disappointed but not discouraged, Rubin persisted. "I didn't have much faith in the test," he says. "I checked with an expert in the field who was of the same opinion. If it's positive, great, but if it's negative, that doesn't necessarily mean anything." Undaunted, Rubin decided to check the ducts himself. Armed with special equipment for culturing actinomycetes, he proceeded to Bradford's building.

That was not the first time Rubin had stepped outside of the ivory tower. As an epidemiology intelligence officer with the CDC, he had chased down hepatitis epidemics, and during the Biafran war in the mid-1960s in Nigeria, he had treated war victims. Once, while investigating a case of rabies in Kansas for the CDC, he helped trap wild animals to track the source of the deadly virus.

So to him, there wasn't anything unusual about shedding his shirt and tie and poking his head into the mouths of the HVAC ducts. He recalls, "We had lunch in the executive dining room first, which was much nicer than the facilities at the hospital. Then I put on work clothes and climbed up a ladder. I took samples and swabs from many areas, especially wet ones."

Next, Rubin planted the material onto culture plates, to see if any thermophilic actinomycetes or other organisms were present. This procedure is similar to a doctor taking a culture from a patient with a possible strep throat. The swab, after being dabbed on a wet surface of a duct in the first case, or on a patient's throat in the second, is then touched to a petri dish that contains nutrients that will support the growth of the microorganism being sought. And sure enough, several days after Rubin obtained the material, an abundant growth of thermophilic actinomycetes was thriving on the plates. Every sample, from every site tested, produced them.

Next, Rubin prepared a new antigen from the bacteria he had obtained in the ducts. He again performed the precipitin test on Bradford's serum, but this time with the new preparation from the ducts at Bradford's office building. Now the precipitin test was strongly positive. There was another unintentional consequence of this phase of the investigation: Bradford inadvertently inhaled another dose of the air from the ducts, and promptly developed mild symptoms again. Another set of x-rays showed a reappearance of the same ominous nodules.

"This clinched the diagnosis," recalls Rubin.

As we continually alter our environment, we create increasing numbers of unnatural hazards. People have developed hypersensitivity pneumonia from central and room humidifiers, heating and cooling systems, moisture-damaged building materials, cool-mist vaporizers, and even automobile air conditioners. One man developed hypersensitivity pneumonia from contaminated water in his home sauna.

Other infectious agents have been transmitted via air-conditioning and ventilation sources, including the bacteria that caused the famous outbreak of Legionnaire's disease at the American Legion convention at the Bellevue-Stratford Hotel in Philadelphia in 1976. In fact, indoor air pollution has become an enormous problem.

The Massachusetts Environmental Protection Agency estimates that 50 percent of all illnesses are attributed to some form of pollution. It further estimates that the annual cost to society is $100 billion, if both medical expenses and worker absenteeism are included.

Some modern office buildings are so contaminated that their occupants suffer from an array of problems—collectively known as the "tight building syndrome" or the "sick building syndrome"—including nasal irritation and nosebleeds, dry throat, scratchy eyes, shortness of breath, lethargy, headache, and more.

The range of contaminants is vast and includes construction dusts, tobacco smoke, and a class of chemicals called volatile organic compounds, which are emitted by copying machines, paints and varnishes, furniture and rugs, and all the other synthetic materials in modern offices. Then there are the organic dusts, like those that caused Bradford's symptoms.

Several studies have shown that workers in buildings with mechanical ventilation—like Bradford's—exhibit many more symptoms than workers in buildings with natural ventilation. In one study, researchers increased the amount of fresh air pumped through a building without telling the workers. Sure enough, the researchers recorded far fewer symptoms of "tight building syndrome" after the increase in ventilation.

Proper ventilation is crucial. In the typical system, fresh outside air is drawn through an intake port. This air is then blown into the building, sometimes after being humidified. The important factor is how often the air is exchanged in these buildings. Fewer air exchanges per day uses less energy and is therefore cheaper, at least in the short run. In industrialized societies, especially in colder climates, people spend a majority of their time indoors, so there is a large potential for this indoor pollution. Proper design of these HVAC systems is important; for example, if the location of the intake port it is too close to traffic, carbon monoxide can be blown into the building.

The magnitude of the problem has been recognized in Massachusetts for some time. In May 1989, the Massachusetts Special Legislative Commission on Indoor Air Pollution issued a report recommending that regulations be strengthened and new legislation be enacted to protect people from these unseen hazards. One expert from Harvard estimated that indoor pollution is the largest public health problem we have and that it could be responsible for as much as 60 to 70 percent of all illnesses.

Dr. Edward Banaszak and his colleagues put it more poetically in the introduction to their report in the *New England Journal of Medicine*. "In classical mythology, the tale of Pandora's box describes how Pandora, in her curiosity, released the evils of the world from a box. The evils were carried forth on winds and breezes to all the world. This early reference to air pollution correlates strikingly with the discovery of hypersensitivity pneumonia due to exposure to a thermophilic actinomycete contaminating a central air-conditioning system."

Once Philip Bradford's problem had been accurately diagnosed, Robert Rubin had one last mystery on his hands. Why hadn't Bradford's fellow office workers also become sick?

"We took serum samples from thirty or forty other workers in the office to look for precipitins, and also inquired about a history of respiratory tract illness," Rubin recalls. "We found five other workers with a high level of antibody similar to Bradford's, with a negative response to the broad-class antigen at the School of Public Health, but a strong [reaction] to the specific antigen derived from the organism isolated from the ductwork. Four of these five co-workers had unexplained respiratory tract disease, which had been diagnosed as 'recurrent pneumonia,' 'weak lungs,' 'smoker's lung,' and a variety of other terms."

Why didn't more workers fall sick? The full answer to this mystery remains elusive, but other building-related clusters of hypersensitivity pneumonia have shown the same phenomenon. Among the possible explanations include an individual's degree of exposure, and differing genetic predispositions, just as some people will develop an allergy to a given exposure while others do not. In the outbreak of hypersensitivity pneumonia from an office air-conditioning system reported by Banaszak, only four of twenty-seven workers developed symptoms, even though all had the same exposure to the air. Of the remaining twenty-three, whose lungs were perfectly normal on pulmonary function testing, eight had positive precipitin tests, but they remained entirely asymptomatic.

After Rubin's investigation, the building's HVAC ducts were thoroughly cleaned, at great expense to its owners. And neither Philip Bradford, who worked in the building for four more years, nor any of his co-workers ever had another bout of the mysterious pneumonia again.

"I am impressed how, in hindsight, we can casually dismiss the possibility of a malignant tumor in this patient. . . . It is remarkable that he escaped a needle biopsy or an open biopsy," said Dr. Wilkins during a clinical case conference that was later held at the Massachusetts General Hospital. "If I get any credit as the patient's first physician at this hospital, it is for picking a detective as well as a physician to take over this diagnostic problem."

~~~~~~~~~~~~~~

Early one afternoon at work, chemical engineer George Melville broke into a sweat, developed pains in his chest, and felt profoundly weak, especially in his thighs. He took himself at once to the emergency room at Lawrence General Hospital in northeastern Massachusetts. A forty-two-year-old male smoker with chest discomfort triggered the usual concern for patient and doctor alike—could this be a heart attack? The usual tests that were available in 1973 were performed. His electrocardiogram (EKG), though strictly speaking abnormal, did not show the clear-cut changes usually found after a heart attack. Blood tests were done. These enzyme tests, which offer supporting evidence in heart attack cases, were also slightly abnormal, but not diagnostic. So far, all of the evidence pointing to a heart attack was circumstantial.

Faced with this ambiguity, the attending physician took the prudent course of action: he ordered Melville (as I'll call him) to be admitted to the intensive care unit for further testing. Over the next day, Melville's doctors tracked down an older EKG taken years before. The "changes" that they were concerned about on his admission EKG had also been present on the earlier recording. And the blood enzyme tests quickly normalized in a pattern not suggesting a heart problem. Analyzing all the evidence that became available during the first two days of the case, his doctors were pretty sure that he did not have a heart attack. Melville also had a low-grade fever and some chills, and although these too are sometimes found after a heart attack, they suggested a whole host of other possible diagnoses as well. The prominent thigh weakness also did not fit with a heart attack. So other tests were done.

This was before HMO medicine and bean counters' scrutiny of "resource utilization." In situations where a diagnosis was unclear, patients would often remain hospitalized simply to have diagnostic testing that in today's medical environment would be undertaken on an outpatient basis. In 1973, Melville stayed in the hospital for two weeks. Even after two weeks of extensive testing, however, his doctors were baffled and the diagnosis remained elusive. Fortunately for Melville, he began feeling fine almost immediately after being admitted. And although they had excluded a heart attack as the cause of the symptoms, the doctors were troubled that they had not a clue about the true nature of his illness. Nevertheless, two weeks after he was admitted, they discharged him home feeling perfectly well.

That might have been the end of the whole affair—except for one curious thing. In conversations around the water cooler, George Melville learned that several of his co-workers had suffered from remarkably similar symptoms. Most had some chest symptoms—usually cough—and many had low-grade fevers. One worker, a twenty-four-year-old supervisor, had three brief but distinct illnesses, each lasting only a day or two. Each episode was nearly identical. He would develop the abrupt onset of weakness, especially in the legs, and a cough, shortness of breath, and wheezing. Each occurrence started in the mid-morning. Twice he consulted his doctor. He too underwent multiple tests, even including a spinal tap; all the results were normal. Ultimately, he was referred to a neurosurgeon, who in turn suggested a psychiatric consultation. He had lots of doctors, but he had no diagnosis.

Two other individuals at Melville's place of work had similar symptoms that on some occasions were severe enough that they had to leave work. One forty-two-year-old woman was hospitalized twice with what was called a "severe viral illness," which sometimes is doctor-speak for "we don't know what's wrong and can't make a specific diagnosis."

George Melville was a manager of a division of Malden Mills, a textile plant with a venerable past situated on the Merrimack River in Lawrence, Massachusetts. The Merrimack, 110 miles long, snakes its way from its origin in Franklin, New Hampshire, to its mouth in Newburyport, Massachusetts, where it empties into the Atlantic. Its powerful current made it an ideal place for factories. In the nineteenth century, because the Merrimack River provided an unending source of power, numerous textile plants sprang up in the area. Malden Mills, which itself has a very colorful history, was one of them. The factory was founded in 1906 by Hungarian immigrant Henry Feuerstein, who worked his way up from sewing blouses in a New York sweatshop to a textile magnate.

The mill's name comes from the fact that the plant was originally located in Malden, Massachusetts.

In 1956, Feuerstein moved Malden Mills to Lawrence, in a complex of red brick buildings along the river's edge. The plant started out making wool sweaters and bathing suits. During World War II, it landed some large government contracts to make fabrics for military use. The textile factory housed all its processes, including dyeing, printing, and finish work, in different buildings on this complex. One early employee in the factory while it was still in Malden was Robert Frost, who grew up in Lawrence. He even wrote a poem, "A Lone Striker," in 1933, that harkens back to his work in the old textile plants.

Like many factories that dot the Merrimack River, Malden Mills houses several of its divisions in brick buildings with large mullioned windows. In its heyday, the plant employed more than three thousand workers. In the particular building where Melville worked, he and thirteen other employees produced imitation crushed velvet, in a process called flocking. The product is one that everyone is more familiar with when it is called velour, which is used in clothing, automobile and home furniture seat covers, novelty items, and other common household accoutrements.

Flock is the industry term for the short fibers that are cut from longer cables of synthetic monofilaments (called tow) that are applied (flocked) onto an adhesive-coated material. In the case of the imitation crushed velvet, the fibers were made of nylon. Because Melville suspected that his illness might have been related to the worksite, he made a telephone call.

Voltaire wrote, "Work keeps us from three great evils: boredom, vice, and need." He was only partly right. Work itself can be an evil; it carries health risks of its own, whether you are a lumberjack in the Pacific Northwest, a fisherman on the Grand Banks off Nova Scotia, or a stock trader on Wall Street.

In 1988, according to the Bureau of Labor Statistics, the private sector reported 6.2 million work-related accidents and nearly a quarter million non-traumatic occupational illnesses, figures that represented substantial increases over previous years. These types of studies often underestimate the frequency of work-related problems. First of all, some occupational illnesses are not detected or recognized as such. Also, exacerbations of chronic illnesses and preexisting diseases by hazardous exposures at work are often not recognized or reported. Furthermore, surveys may not include small businesses, which, combined, employ large numbers of workers. One statistic that is less ambiguous is job-related deaths; there were 3,270 of them in 1988.

Occupational medicine was largely ignored by the medical community until the 1980s. Over the past decade, demand for expertise has risen sharply because of increasing governmental regulation, litigation stemming from toxic exposures, and mounting public recognition of environmental risks. Two federal agencies that were created in 1970, the National Institute for Occupational Safety and Health (NIOSH) and the Occupational Safety and Health Administration (OSHA), police American industry. NIOSH is the research and advisory branch, investigating potential work-related disease outbreaks and performing industry-wide surveys. It advises OSHA, which writes the standards, inspects workplaces for compliance, and enforces the standards by imposing fines.

When Melville fell sick in 1973, however, expertise was hard to come by. Fortunately, he lived in an area where help was just a phone call away. Harvard's School of Public Health, he thought, would surely be able to help find an explanation.

"I received a call one day from this man, asking us to investigate what he thought was a problem with his plant," recalls John Peters, then an associate professor of occupational medicine at the Harvard School of Public Health (and now a professor of occupational and environmental medicine at the University of Southern California School of Medicine). "He [Melville] told me about his hospitalization and then about a couple of other people with vague symptoms, one of whom had been hospitalized twice for what was thought to be a severe viral illness," recalls Peters. "Another guy had a couple of attacks which he had attributed to the work setting. On that basis, he wanted me to get involved. So I did.

"I visited the textile mill to figure out the process, understand all the elements and possible exposures." This is a standard occupational health approach to a possible outbreak of disease in the workplace. The investigators generally follow a three-step plan. First, understand the details of the process—the workflow. Often a change has been instituted recently that may seem very minor to the employees or to the bosses, so it goes unnoticed. Second, using this detailed analysis of the workflow process, generate a list of possible exposures. Last, interview the workers and tabulate the information, in standard epidemiologist fashion, to see if any clues fall out.

So this is what Peters, and his colleague Dr. David Wegman, did. They talked with the thirteen men and women, ages nineteen to sixty-one, who worked with Melville. Some had been employed in the velvet flocking division for as long as six years. The investigators learned from the managers of Malden Mills, who were very cooperative, that the process for making the crushed velvet had been changed recently, and that the workers' health complaints had started after the introduction of the new manufacturing process.

The odd thing was that only seven of the thirteen workers were experiencing problems. Dr. Peters conducted detailed interviews with all of them. A prevailing story emerged from these discussions.

"It was so standard," he says, "that I thought these people must have been talking to one another and rehearsing. Of course, they hadn't been. They would report to work feeling fine, and then they would develop a typical sequence of symptoms." Most had a cough with fever or chills. Many complained of weakness and achy pains throughout their body; a few suffered from shortness of breath. Melville had experienced chest pain. The symptoms would develop at work and last an average of twenty-four hours. The workers would never get the symptoms on weekends.

In this kind of analysis, what does not happen can be just as important as what did happen, like the dog that didn't bark in the Sherlock Holmes story *The Hound of the Baskervilles*. Why did six of the workers never get sick? The reason could not be explained on the basis of age or sex or any other obvious variables. They all worked in the same division in the same building and therefore had the same exposures. So Peters examined the manufacturing process in detail, hoping to find a clue about why some workers were affected and others were not.

In the flocking process at the plant, nylon fibers were first dyed and then cut into short strips measuring about an eighth of an inch. Next, they were treated with a clay slurry to facilitate their forming a velvety pattern when fixed to a rayon cloth. The flocking step involved treating the cloth with an adhesive and a formaldehyde resin to fix the nylon fibers onto the rayon surface. The material was then cured at 300–330 degrees Fahrenheit, using ammonia to stabilize the acidity.

After flocking, some of the material, about 20 percent, was used in a different process that involved different employees, so this part of the routine fell outside the investigators' analysis. The remaining 80 percent was treated with a fluorocarbon polymer to make it stain resistant and waterproof. Next it was dipped, rolled, and squeezed, then cured at 300–310 degrees, and finally crushed and steamed at 275 degrees. Last, the crushed velvet was cooled, back-steamed at 190 degrees, and then treated to eliminate static electricity. This last step could potentially produce ozone.

"So there were several potential exposures," says Peters, "but there were problems with all of them. We looked for ozone but didn't find any. And both the ammonia and the formaldehyde were present in too low a concentration to be toxic. Plus, the nylon fibers were too large to be inhaled into the lungs." That left the fluorocarbon polymer. There were several hints that it might be the source of the problem. For one, none of the workers who handled the cloth that had not been treated with the polymer ever got sick. Second, the rest of the workers rotated jobs, and these workers got sick only when they did handle the polymer-treated cloth. And last, Peters was aware of a syndrome called polymer-fume fever, an illness that matched the textile workers' symptoms perfectly.

The word "polymer" derives from the Greek *poly* (many) and *meros* (part). Polymers consist of simple substances linked chemically in long chains, with the resulting structure having properties different from those of the individual components. The polymer used in the crushed velvet flocking process is called polytetrafluoroethylene, mercifully referred to as PTFE.

The history of PTFE in itself is remarkable. Like many other important discoveries, PTFE was stumbled upon completely by accident. A research chemist named Roy Plunkett, working for the DuPont Company in the late 1930s, was searching for a better refrigerant. Early refrigerants, such as ammonia and sulfur dioxide, regularly poisoned food-industry workers and even people in their homes. In his search for a safer method, he was working with tetrafluoroethyelene (TFE). At normal temperatures, TFE is a gas, and Plunkett had prepared hundred-pound cylinders of TFE in preparation for adding chlorine. To keep the gas stable overnight, he froze some of the metal tanks in dry ice. The next morning, April 6, 1938, he opened one of the tanks, but nothing came out.

Thinking that the gas must have escaped, he weighed the tank to test that hypothesis (since a full tank would weigh more than an empty tank). The weight showed that none of the gas had escaped. Plunkett and his assistant sawed open the tank and found that it contained a white waxy solid that on further analysis turned out to be polymerized TFE—or PTFE. Curious about this new substance, Plunkett experimented with it further and found that it had amazing heat resistance and was chemically inert; that is, it would not react with other substances. In addition, one of its most important qualities was its low surface friction, so low that almost nothing stuck to it. The first scientific report on PTFE was published in 1941.

For all of these reasons, Plunkett and DuPont realized that there were probably some commercial uses for PTFE. They began using it in many other applications, but one of the first general uses for it was in 1946 when it was used to coat cookware to prevent food from sticking. The company needed a trade name and came up with a rather catchy one: Teflon.

Within ten years of the 1941 report however, the first cases of toxicity surfaced. D. Kenwin Harris was a divisional medical officer in the plastics industry in England. He wrote an article that was published in the medical journal *The Lancet*, titled "Polymer-Fume Fever," in 1951. This terse report contains quite a bit of information that had a direct bearing on the investigation at Malden Mills.

The description Harris gave remains remarkably accurate. He wrote:

> *There is always a latent period, often of a few hours between the original exposure to the fume and the development of symptoms. People who are unaware of the hazard sometimes think that they are developing a cold or influenza, and then to attribute their symptoms to this, especially as the*

illness may not start until they have finished work and gone home. The rapid recovery tends to confirm their belief; hence, it is not uncommon for employees not to seek assistance until they have had more than one attack.

The first symptom is a sense of discomfort in the chest, especially on taking a deep breath. This may be a feeling of irritation or oppression behind the sternum, but is never severe enough to warrant the words "pain" or "constriction" and often the patient has some difficulty in describing it. The patient may or may not develop a dry irritating cough, which becomes worse with the gradual increase of soreness in the chest.

He went on to say: "Physical signs are notable for their evanescence or complete absence. . . . An acute attack subsides quickly, and within a day or two at the most, the patient has completely recovered."

Dr. Harris went on to describe two clinical cases of polymer-fume fever and referenced two others described from a doctor associated with the DuPont chemical company. He pursued the matter further by doing some experiments on rats. He exposed these laboratory animals to PTFE in order to further elucidate the cause of the symptoms. The results of those experiments showed that temperature was a critical factor. At temperatures below 570 degrees F, the polymer seemed stable and did not emit any of the toxic fumes.

This was not the first time the fumes from an industrial material were found to be the culprit in human disease. Metal-fume fever was first described by a Dr. Potissier in 1822. Brass workers developed similar symptoms, leading to the terms "brass founders' ague" and "brass fever." Many of these syndromes related to inhalation of microscopic particles of the oxides of various metals, including copper, zinc, magnesium, and many others. When these metals are being welded (such as in ship building) or melted or smelted, particles thirty times smaller than a single red blood cell are released into the air. When workers breathe this material into their lungs, they can develop the same symptoms that George Melville and his co-workers had. In these older reports, some patients had fevers so high as to suggest the diagnosis of malaria.

In spite of this long and colorful history, Peters still had two big problems with the otherwise logical hypothesis that the polymer was causing the illnesses. First, not all of the workers exposed to the polymer got sick. And, more important, it is not the polymer itself that causes the syndrome; it is the fumes produced when the polymer is heated above 570 degrees. The highest recorded temperature in the crushed velvet manufacturing process was 330 degrees.

"So we were sort of stuck," recalls Peters. It kept coming back to the same question: Why did some of the workers have it, and others not? When Peters reanalyzed the information from the interviews, the answer was as simple as it was (at least in retrospect) obvious. "I got lucky. Because of the prominent respiratory symptoms, we included a question on the questionnaire about cigarette smoking. That turned out to be the clue in the end."

Most of the workers who developed polymer-fume fever were smokers. Melville smoked a pipe. Employees using the polymer handled and adjusted the cloth as it was dipped, rolled, squeezed, and cured, thus contaminating their hands with the PTFE. The flow of work also allowed for frequent breaks, during which the workers often smoked cigarettes without first washing their hands. The association of cigarette smoking and polymer-fume fever had been made before. In 1963, a report making this connection came out in the *Transactions of the Association of Industrial Medical Officers*, an arcane publication that would not have been available to the average physician.

In 1965, another, much larger report of an epidemic of thirty-six workers at a large industrial plant in Kansas was reported in the (far more prominent) *Journal of the American Medical Association*. The details in this case had a number of similarities to the goings-on at Malden Mills. Workers in an assembly plant were affected—but not all of them. The start of the epidemic coincided with two changes in the work flow. The first involved the use of a new parting compound that used PTFE, and the second related to decreased ventilation in that area of the plant with the advent of a new air-conditioning unit. Most of the sick workers smoked, and the remainder of them were using an air gun that heated the air to 750 degrees Fahrenheit, well above the critical temperature at which PTFE becomes toxic. Fixing the ventilation and forbidding smoking in the plant were the only steps required to halt the outbreak.

In 1972, other physicians published a report about the unusual case of a fifty-year-old woman with polymer-fume fever. She had more than forty attacks over a nine-month period before the true cause was established. She smoked a pack a day. A female co-worker who had the same exposure, but was a nonsmoker, remained well. So there was precedent in the medical literature for the connection between polymer-fume fever and smoking.

How hot could a cigarette be, though? After all, it doesn't burn the smoker. One group of researchers found that the average temperature in the combustion zone of a cigarette is about 1620 degrees F—nearly three times the temperature required to produce toxic fumes from the polymer. But how much PTFE would be necessary on the fingers of the workers to produce enough of the fume to lead to illness? One study of human volunteers found that the disease can occur with as little as 0.4 milligrams of PTFE. Another researcher, R. J. Sherwood, discovered that a substantial concentration of fumes is achieved by smoking a cigarette contaminated with a piece of polymer the size of a grain of sand.

Once the problem at the Lawrence textile mill was clearly defined, the solution proved quite simple. The workplace was designated a no-smoking area, and no one was allowed to smoke or eat without first washing his or her hands. No further cases of polymer-fume fever occurred.

End of story, right?

Not exactly.

First of all, outbreaks of polymer-fume fever continued to crop up from time to time. Over a nine-month period from July 1985 to March 1986, three workers from a Mississippi sign and stamp manufacturing shop had repeated episodes of a severe "flu-like illness" with prominent muscle and back pain. The workers would develop these same symptoms a few times per week but never on weekends. Only the workers making rubber and metal stamps were affected.

After months of this pattern, the company's owner finally asked NIOSH to evaluate the situation. In a series of events remarkably similar to those found at Malden Mills, the investigators learned that the owners had recently made a change in the process. In July 1985, the company had started making its stamps using a new asbestos-free board for its molds. After the workers poured the rubber into the mold board, they baked the board in a small oven that reached 580 degrees F. But at the last step of the process, the rubber stamps tended to stick to the new board, so the workers started using a mold-release spray, to help the stamps come free from the board. The supplier of this spray, which included a fluorocarbon as a trace ingredient, did not include the possibility of polymer-fume fever in its safety sheet. As in previous outbreaks, as soon as the problem was clear, a simple solution was implemented and no further illness was reported.

A second incident related to the nylon flock industry went beyond medicine and took on decidedly political and ethical overtones. In 1990, a man working for a company called Microfibers, Incorporated, saw his doctor in Ontario, Canada, because of shortness of breath and a cough. His specific job at Microfibers was making flock. He was ultimately diagnosed with interstitial lung disease, a relatively rare condition in which the lung becomes inflamed and can scar. This sometimes results in chronic breathing problems severe enough to require oxygen therapy twenty-four hours a day. When other workers at the same plant were similarly afflicted, and one nearly died of it, the Canadian government implemented changes to prevent the disease.

Four years later, in November 1994, a textile worker at a Microfibers plant in Pawtucket, Rhode Island, developed similar symptoms and was also found to have interstitial lung disease. The patient was referred to an occupational health specialist, Dr. David Kern. He visited the plant and, contrary to the cooperative spirit at Malden Mills, he recalls, "At the door, we were greeted by the personnel director, who asked us to sign a trade secret confidentiality agreement." Kern signed the document and began his investigation, which was similar in tactics to those used by Peters in the Malden Mills affair. He found nothing suspicious and concluded that this was likely not an occupational issue.

But when a second worker from the same plant was referred to him about a year later, in January 1996, Kern began to rethink the issue. Finding two cases of a rare disease in patients who worked at the same plant suggested a relationship and a possible occupational cause. The company also requested a NIOSH investigation, and Kern launched a parallel inquiry. When Kern tested all of the 165 textile workers at the plant, he found that 7 of them had the same findings; the incidence of interstitial lung disease was an astonishing 50 times higher than that in the general population. This was big news, so in 1996, while these two investigations were ongoing, Kern planned to present some of the preliminary information as an abstract at the 1997 meeting of the American Thoracic Society.

An abstract is usually a brief report of early work that is not quite ready to be formally published in a medical journal. Its purpose is to alert other doctors and scientists about preliminary findings. Sometimes doctors at professional meetings will read abstracts and find other researchers who are working on the same problem, and this can facilitate collaboration. It is such a standard academic practice that Kern was surprised when the textile company asked him not to submit the abstract. A company spokesman argued that the abstract included proprietary information and that it would therefore violate the confidentiality agreement that Kern had signed two years earlier. Kern was flabbergasted that an agreement he had signed in 1994 was being applied to an investigation that he had not even started until 1995.

Once again, the nylon flock appeared to be the culprit. But unlike the transient symptoms that are seen with polymer-fume fever, this new group of patients seemed to have permanent damage to the lungs. He was concerned about the development of a previously unrecognized syndrome resulting in permanent damage to the lungs. Furthermore some cases resulted in severe lung damage; one patient had needed to be on a ventilator in the ICU and nearly died. Kern was also worried because this new syndrome was occurring in an industry with approximately twenty-five hundred employees in the United States and many thousands more worldwide. New cases were surfacing as more time elapsed and Kern investigated more thoroughly. Because the syndrome was almost certainly preventable, Kern wanted to broadcast it as loudly as possible.

That is when the situation turned even uglier. Kern's occupational health clinic was at Memorial Hospital in Pawtucket, and he maintained a faculty post at Brown University School of Medicine. Lawyers became involved. Brown University threatened to fire him. The hospital warned him that it might shut down his occupational health unit. Kern countersued the university, the hospital, and Microfibers, claiming that his rights under the Occupational Safety and Health Act had been violated. Kern's friends and colleagues began a letter-writing campaign. One week after he presented his abstract in the spring of 1997, both the hospital and the university sent Kern letters informing him that his five-year contract would not be renewed. Numerous counterclaims were made. More than seventy occupational physicians supported Kern, in part referring to the history of asbestosis, another product of a toxic substance once thought to be safe. They invoked "the obligation to report."

In the end, Kern and colleagues published their findings in the *Annals of Internal Medicine*, and a new term was coined—flock worker's lung. Their article, which appeared in 1998, described a cause of chronic interstitial lung disease that had never been previously reported. The paper detailed eight cases that were related not to the polymer PTFE but to the nylon fibers themselves, which, it turns out, can enter the respiratory tract and cause inflammation. The following year, NIOSH sponsored a workshop for clinicians dedicated to studying this new entity.

The final episode involving flock exposure brings the story full circle. This one goes back to the same problem George Melville had—polymer-fume fever—and, remarkably enough, the same place, Malden Mills.

Malden Mills continued to reinvent itself as a company. It went bankrupt in 1981, but the company came roaring back with a new synthetic fabric called Polarfleece, made from a polyester fiber that wicks moisture away from the body. In the 1980s and 1990s, the fabric and its second generation—Polartec—became immensely popular with various high-end outdoor clothing manufacturers. Demand for its imitation velvet fabric for home furnishings also grew, and the company emerged from bankruptcy in 1983. Business soared by 200 percent, and Malden Mills became a $3 billion company. By 1986, sales were so strong that the company began investing $10 million per year in state-of-the-art research, design, and production equipment to keep up with the ever-growing demand for its products. Such big-name outfits as Patagonia, Lands End, Eddie Bauer, L. L. Bean, and others were buying up as much fabric as Malden Mills could produce.

In the 1990s, Malden Mills stood out as one of the few textile manufacturers that was able to survive the stringent environmental laws and high labor costs in Massachusetts. As if the company itself had a soul, it launched initiatives to protect the environment by building a water treatment plant to restore the Merrimack River systems around the company's mills. It reduced the amount of chemicals necessary to manufacture its products. It worked to conserve energy and reduce waste. The company had an ever-growing international market for its products.

Then on December 11, 1995, as Aaron Feuerstein was celebrating his seventieth birthday, an explosion rocked the plant and caused a fire that destroyed three of the nine buildings. Feuerstein, a grandson of the original founder and by this time the company's CEO, vowed to rebuild. In a move that shocked many in the business world, he even continued to pay the out-of-work employees for as long as funds held out. The move sparked such notoriety that President Bill Clinton mentioned it in his State of the Union address in January 1996.

Since then, the company has again been in bankruptcy and again emerged from it, in 2003, this time without the Feuerstein family at the helm. The Lawrence plant is home to about a thousand workers in the new century.

But Malden Mills is still a plant, and as such it is no less vulnerable to industrial illnesses. The last part of the story shows the importance of institutional memory.

"Several years after the outbreak of polymer-fume fever," recalls Peters, "a few of us at Harvard had started a consulting firm to deal with health problems in industry, and we got a call one day from this same plant [Malden Mills], where workers were once again experiencing similar difficulties. There were different people working there now, and they had done something funny over the weekend. Somehow, they had gotten the polymer into the heating system. There was an odd weather pattern on the next Monday, so that wind was blowing from an unusual direction, forcing the exhaust from the heating system back into the building through the ventilation intakes.

"There were a number of cases and, sure enough, they were all clustered around the ventilation intake ports. We solved this one by altering the ventilation system." And since then, Malden Mills has not had any further problems with polymer-fume fever.

9 The Case of the Wide-Eyed Boy

~~~~~~~~~~~~~~~~~~~~~~~~~~~~~

Although Gary Setnik had been a specialist in emergency medicine for fifteen years, he's still never sure what to expect. On any given day at Mount Auburn Hospital in Cambridge, Massachusetts, he may see a child with the sniffles, a teenager with a seizure, a grandmother with pneumonia, or an executive in cardiac arrest. As time passes, the details of many of those cases blur into one another.

But doctors will recall the smallest details of some cases even years later.

"In spite of the fact that you see thousands of patients, there are a very few cases that stand out as being so unusual and so rewarding that they become part of your foremost memories," Setnik says, settling back in his leather chair in his Cambridge office to recall one of them. "And this is certainly one of those cases.

"It was a cloudy Sunday afternoon in October, a few years ago, around 1985 or so. I very clearly remember going to the chart rack, picking up the record of the next patient, and being immediately struck by the information available."

The chart belonged to a ten-year-old boy I'll call Shawn Matthews. A triage nurse, usually the first person to interact with a new patient in an emergency department, had already made some notations on Shawn's chart. The young boy's chief complaints, according to the nurse, were headache and blurred vision. She recorded his vital signs, which were remarkable only in that they were completely normal, and then pointed out that Shawn's left pupil was markedly dilated. This was the information that Setnik had available at that moment.

"Before I even stepped away from the chart rack," recalls Setnik, the chairman of the department of emergency medicine at Mount Auburn, "I was considering all the possible causes of headache and dilated pupil. Most of them were bad. So it was with some urgency that I walked into the room and introduced myself. I can even recall the specific room; it was 11-R. Shawn was sitting on the examination table, with his parents and a younger sister clustered around. I instantly noticed the asymmetry of his pupils. The right one was normal, but the left one filled the entire iris, the colored part of the eye. Shawn appeared well, was breathing normally and didn't seem to be in any pain. He was a little anxious, but no more so than any other ten-year-old whose parents had brought him to an emergency room.

"I turned to the parents and started asking questions. Mr. Matthews said that, other than some ear infections as a toddler, Shawn had always been in excellent health and seemed entirely well until shortly after breakfast, when he began complaining of a headache behind his left eye and blurred vision. When he told his parents, they noticed the dilated pupil and promptly brought him to the emergency room. There was no history of eye injury or trauma, medications, use of eye drops, or any past or family history of eye problems. He had no fever, stiff neck, and so on."

Next, Setnik questioned Shawn directly. The boy told him that the headache was constant and dull, and located directly behind the abnormal eye. Shawn had no problem speaking, chewing, swallowing, or walking, and no difficulty with balance. He had been playing in his room when the headache began, but nothing unusual had occurred.

Before examining Shawn, Setnik began to consider what lay ahead. "I wondered if he was going to need other, sophisticated tests and the expertise of a pediatric neurosurgeon. The mind of an emergency physician is always moving two or three steps ahead, time being of the essence. One thing that distinguishes emergency medicine from many other specialties is that time is such a major component in the management of the patient. I was already thinking, will I need to transfer this boy to a hospital with a pediatric neurosurgeon? Would he require an ambulance or would I let the parents drive him in the family car? Initially, I had two possible concerns. The first possible cause of Shawn's symptoms was eye trauma, but there was no history of that. The other possibility that came to mind, and the one that I was most concerned about, was could this be an aneurysm of a cerebral artery."

The eye is one of the body's great marvels, and the iris is a wonder in itself. The pupil of the eye is the dark central area that is surrounded by the colored part, the iris. The iris is actually the business portion of the apparatus that continually adjusts the size of the pupil, which is essentially just a hole in the iris. Although we usually take this mechanism for granted, imagine stepping out of a darkened movie theater into bright sunshine. The importance of the iris's never-ending task becomes instantly apparent. In the dim light of the theater, dilator muscles in the iris contract, dilating the pupil and allowing more light to strike the retina, so that we can see better in the darkness. This mechanism operates on the same principle as the aperture setting of a camera. As you walk out of the darkened theater, the sunlight floods the retina with too much light for your dilated pupils. You automatically squint and raise your hand to shade your eyes. But within seconds, the sphincter muscles of the iris constrict, making the pupil smaller and allowing less light into the eye.

The pupil continually adjusts and readjusts, depending on both the brightness and the distance of the object that you're looking at. Generally, both pupils are the same size, but in up to 25 percent of normal individuals, small differences in pupillary size may occur intermittently and occasionally even switch sides from one to the other.

The nervous system, just as it does for all the muscles in the body, controls the iris. And, as with all of the body's involuntary muscles, those responsible for bodily functions that we do not consciously think about (like the heart or intestine or diaphragm), it is the autonomic nervous system that regulates the size of the pupils. The autonomic nervous system consists of two parts—the sympathetic and the parasympathetic components. These are like the yin and yang of the body. The sympathetic system gears the body for action—accelerated heartbeat, increased rate of breathing, diminished intestinal activity and salivary secretions—known as the fight-or-flight response. The parasympathetic system does the opposite. It increases salivary secretions, augments intestinal activity, and slows the heart and respiratory rates. As for pupil size, the sympathetic nervous system dilates and the parasympathetic constricts. Like yin and yang, these two components of the autonomic nervous system are continually establishing balance with each other and setting the right tone for any given situation.

There are other differences in the way that the sympathetics and parasympathetics affect the eye; one of those differences is the route taken by the nerve fibers to get to the eye. The sympathetic fibers originate in the thoracic portion of the spinal cord, regroup in a ganglion in the neck, and then hitch a ride along blood vessels to find their way to the iris. The parasympathetic fibers come from deep in the midbrain, a primitive part of the brainstem, then exit the brain as part of the third cranial nerve. This nerve, which includes other fibers that control eye movements, courses along the floor of the skull to find its way to the orbit. As it exits the brain, it enters what is known as the subarachnoid space, the area where the cerebrospinal fluid resides. This clear fluid supplies nutrients to the brain and spinal cord and acts as a shock absorber as well. As the third cranial nerve traverses this fluid-filled space, it is vulnerable to compression by other structures in the region. One of those structures is the posterior communicating artery, a blood vessel that links up the arterial supply in the front of the brain with that of the back (posterior) part. If something were to press on the nerve in this location, then the yin and yang would be thrown out of balance. In this case, the mass could push on the parasympathetic fibers, and diminish their function. The sympathetics, because of their different path to the eye, would remain active and unopposed, resulting in a dilated pupil.

With knowledge of this anatomy in mind, and noting normal findings on Shawn's throat, neck, heart, lung, and abdominal examination, Setnik turned his attention to the boy's nervous system. He checked Shawn's sensation, strength, balance, and reflexes. He listened over his skull for bruits (French for noises)—whooshing sounds caused by a tangle of abnormal cerebral blood vessels. He inspected the retina with an ophthalmoscope, looking for signs of brain swelling or bleeding. He checked Shawn's neck for stiffness, an indicator of inflammation in the subarachnoid space.

"I very carefully checked the movements of his eyes, because the same nerve that controls the pupils also controls some eye motions. His eyes moved completely normally," recalls Setnik. "I checked all of the twelve cranial nerves and I did a detailed pupil exam. When you shine a light in one pupil, both of them will constrict; that's called the consensual reaction. The dilated pupil did not react. The pupil will also constrict when a person switches from looking at an object in the distance to looking at a near object; that's called the accommodation reflex. His dilated pupil did not constrict to near objects either." But except for the dilated pupil, Shawn seemed to be perfectly healthy.

It didn't add up.

"At the end of that examination, I sat back and I remember putting my fingers to my bearded chin and just thinking. I was struck by how well he looked. It was just my gut feeling that he wasn't sick. You develop this instinct as an emergency physician; it's not very scientific but you get pretty good at it. There are times when you don't act reflexively but you just sit down and give yourself space to think. I was confronted now by a most unusual situation. It was becoming less conceivable to me that the likeliest diagnosis—bleeding or pressure on a nerve—was really the problem. Bottom line is that Shawn just didn't look sick to me. Also, his eye movements were normal, and I thought that it would be unusual for the pupil to be dilated from a nerve lesion without any effect on the muscles that move the eyes."

Setnik knew all too well that a relatively common mass that can compress the third cranial nerve is an aneurysm of the posterior communicating artery. Aneurysms are outpouchings in a weak spot of an artery. Like a weak spot in a tire that balloons out from the pressure of the air within, aneurysms can balloon out from an artery under the pressure of blood. They can occur in any artery of the body. Aneurysms in and around the brain are surprisingly common; they occur in up to 2 percent of people. In most cases, they never cause symptoms and are never detected. But for reasons that are not completely understood, in some patients they begin to grow. Sometimes, when they grow large enough, they will rupture. When they do, patients usually have an excruciating pain, the worst headache of their life. Because these aneurysms are almost always in the subarachnoid space, this bleeding is known as a subarachnoid hemorrhage. It is usually diagnosed with a CT scan or by a lumbar puncture, or spinal tap.

After experiencing a subarachnoid hemorrhage, patients must be treated very quickly. In the late 1980s, when this case occurred, the primary treatment was open brain surgery. The first step would be to carry out an angiogram to identify an aneurysm and then rapidly perform a procedure to isolate it from the circulation and protect the patient from further bleeding. At the time Setnik saw Shawn Matthews, the angiogram itself had some risk. A doctor would insert a catheter into the femoral artery in the groin and snake it up the aorta and into the major arteries of the brain. The patient would be injected with a small amount of dye, and then x-rays would be taken. The dye would show the outlines of the arteries in the brain, and if there was an aneurysm, it would appear in the x-ray. Once the aneurysm was defined, a specially trained neurosurgeon would drill holes into the skull and remove a flap of bone to expose the brain. The surgeon would carefully retract portions of the brain to expose the major blood vessel that includes the aneurysm. The surgeon would place a metal clamp across the base of the aneurysm, thus excluding it from the rest of the circulation and preventing any subsequent rupture.

Nowadays, there are much less invasive aneurysm treatments called endovascular therapy. A physician with special training will place a platinum coil inside the aneurysm via a catheter similar to the one used for the angiogram. The coils induce the blood in the aneurysm to clot, which functionally excludes the aneurysm from the circulation the same as surgery.

Aneurysms don't always present with a subarachnoid hemorrhage, however. Sometimes they expand but do not rupture. If the aneurysm happens to be on the posterior communicating artery, it often presses on the third cranial nerve. When it does, the pupil dilates and there is often a mild headache. If Setnik's worst fears were true, Shawn might need to be transported to a specialized pediatric neurosurgical center for an angiogram and brain surgery.

"At that point, I recalled another patient I had seen about five years previously. He was a Harvard grad student who had been working in a chemistry lab and came in with a dilated pupil too. The chemical he was working with was atropine, which is a potent stimulus for pupillary dilation. That man had accidentally gotten some on his finger, then causally rubbed his eye. Somehow, the two cases linked up in my mind."

Atropine has a long and checkered past. It is an alkaloid, extracted from an herb native to Europe and Asia that produces sweet black berries. Botanists call it *Atropa belladonna;* its common name is deadly nightshade or devil's cherries. The plant is widely distributed and can be found across large parts of central and southern Europe, southwestern Asia, Algeria, and North America. A bushy plant that grows several feet high, it prefers the shade beneath large trees. The leaves are a dull dark green of various sizes between three and ten inches in length. The dull purple flowers appear in June and July, and bloom through September, at which time they form a black berry about the size of a small cherry. These berries contain a dark, inky juice that is seductively sweet.

The herb belongs to the Solanacea family, a very large group of plants that contains some members that are quite edible and others that are incredibly toxic to humans. Such important staples of the human food supply as tomatoes, eggplants, chili and Tabasco peppers, and potatoes belong to the Solanacea family. So does the petunia. And so does the tobacco plant, from which the alkaloid nicotine is derived. Nicotine has many effects on humans—some toxic, others physiologic.

As entrenched in the human food chain as the potato is now, it was not always so. The potato probably originated in the Chilean Andes thirteen thousand years ago and was not cultivated in the area until five thousand years later. When the Spanish encountered the potato in the late sixteenth century, they did not welcome it at all. One reason was that the potato was a plant without standard growing seasons that the Europeans were accustomed to. The other reason was that Europeans thought the potato plant too closely resembled other plants that Western society had feared for millennia.

Consider the henbane plant. This herb is indigenous to many parts of Europe and Asia and has been imported to the New World. Its leaves, which are of medicinal value, have been harvested for over two thousand years. Its two major alkaloids, hyoscyamine and scopolamine, have important pharmacologic effects on humans. Henbane will commonly induce hallucinations, dilated pupils, restlessness, and flushed skin. The Egyptian queen Cleopatra is rumored to have used an extract of the plant to kill her enemies, although when she decided to end her own life she settled on a bite from an asp. She also recognized that a much more dilute solution, when placed in the eyes, would dilate her pupils to make her more alluring. Henbane's effects were also known to the ancient Greeks and Romans. The priestess of Apollo allegedly used it to help increase the accuracy of her pronouncements. In the Middle Ages, criminals used an extract of henbane as a poison. It was also used in traditional German pilsner beers until 1516, when the Bavarian Purity Law abolished its use in favor of a brew made from pure hops.

Another poisonous plant from the Solanacea group is the datura. This foul-smelling plant originated in India but has spread all over the world. Some believe that it first reached North America at Jamestown, Virginia, because records suggest that sailors in the original settlement were poisoned by it. After eating it like spinach, they nearly died. This led to the name Jamestown weed, which at some point became contracted to simply jimsonweed. During the Middle Ages, Italian professional killers devised a brew from the datura plant that not only would kill those who drank it, but had the advantage (to the criminal) of dulling the victims' senses before they died. Extracts from this plant have a decided psychogenic effect. Hindu prostitutes in the sixteenth century used it to dope their clients, and white slavers were reputed to use it as an aphrodisiac.

The major plant in this group, and the one with the most significance for humans, is the deadly nightshade, *Atropa belladonna*, a plant with a double-edged history as both a poison and a medication. The genus name, *Atropa*, derives from Atropos, the oldest of the three fates, and the one that was responsible for snipping the thread of life. So, as the name implies, atropine is deadly. Eating a single berry can be fatal.

The plant has influenced several military campaigns. Belladonna was allegedly the poison that weakened Marc Antony's troops during the Parthian Wars. According to Plutarch, "Those who sought for herbs obtained few that they had been accustomed to eat, and in tasting unknown herbs, they found one that brought on madness and death. He that had eaten of it immediately lost all memory and knowledge, but at the same time would busy himself in turning and moving every stone he met with, as if he was upon some very important pursuit. The camp was full of unhappy men, bending to the ground and thus digging up and removing stones, till at last they were carried off by a bilious vomiting, when wine, the only remedy, was not to be found."

The Scottish army under Macbeth used belladonna to poison the Danish troops during a "truce." The Scots supplied the Danes with liquor that had been infused with a root that was likely belladonna. This escapade finds its way into Shakespeare's *Macbeth*, when Banquo says, "Or have we eaten of the insane root that takes the reason prisoner?"

It's more than a poison, though. Women in Renaissance Italy learned what Cleopatra had known about henbane. If they applied a very dilute drop of the plant's juice to their eyes, it would make the pupils dilate, thus enhancing the user's beauty. Hence, the species name—*belladonna*, Italian for "beautiful lady."

The berries appear similar enough to those of edible species that people sometimes eat them by mistake. The *Lancet* in 1846 chronicled the case of an herbalist who was hawking his wares in the Whitechapel Road area. A woman bought a pint of so-called nettleberries for three pence and made a pie. The journal reported: "Her husband ate more heartily of the pie than she did. Before the remains of the dinner were removed, a customer came in to pay some money, and was accompanied by a child, named Samuel Jones. The little boy looked very anxiously at the tart, and she gave him some, little thinking at that time that the berries were poisonous. A few minutes after her husband had finished his dinner, he said he was very drowsy, and went into the bar-parlour. His lethargy soon increased, his countenance changed colour, and the pupils of his eyes became dilated. He said he had a very strange coppery taste in his mouth, and that he would go up stairs and lie down upon the bed. As he went up stairs he staggered, and upon entering his bedroom fell upon the floor, and became insensible." By the next morning, both the man and the little boy were dead, and several others who had eaten the berries had fallen seriously ill.

There were also medical uses for belladonna. As of 1803, it was still used to treat febrile illnesses such as plague, apoplexy, whooping cough, rabies, depression, and mania. Nineteenth-century practitioners were aware of the toxic properties and recommended gradually increasing the dose from day to day, until the patient developed "tension in the throat," a sign of toxicity.

In the mid-nineteenth century, medicinal chemistry was becoming a well-developed science, and chemists from France, Germany, and Britain were all busy in their labs trying to uncover the secrets of the human nervous system and the various plants that had been used for centuries. In 1831, a German apothecary was the first to isolate atropine from the roots of the belladonna plant. These discoveries helped physiologists unravel the components of the autonomic nervous system.

Atropine, sometimes marketed as belladonna on the label, was used for neuralgia, back pain and joint complaints, tuberculosis, and a variety of other conditions. It was incorporated into bandages to help heal skin lesions. So even though the science was evolving, the use of atropine was anything but scientific. In part because of this, atropine poisoning was a regular occurrence as the nineteenth century became the twentieth.

So common was it that in 1911, a physician collected reports of 682 cases of atropine poisoning, 60 of whom died. Of the total, 379 were accidental cases caused by the use of belladonna eye drops, bandages, and salves, and another 303 were from the pure alkaloid. However, 37 were suicides, and 14 were deemed to be murders.

The symptoms of atropine poisoning result from an imbalance in the autonomic nervous system. Patients often have hallucinations; many can be seen muttering unintelligibly or picking at invisible objects in their clothes or bed sheets. They tend to be agitated and restless. Their gait is unstable. In short, they can appear intoxicated by alcohol. Their pulse is quick and their temperature is often elevated. The skin is dry and sometimes appears red. Doctors have a mnemonic for this classic cluster of symptoms—"hot as a hare, blind as a bat, dry as a bone, red as a beet, and mad as a hatter."

The "blind as a bat" refers to the effects of atropine on the eye; it dilates the pupil, sometimes so much that there is no iris left to see. Atropine also reduces the ability of the iris to accommodate to changes in ambient light and distance. This results in blurry vision.

A synthetic atropine-like drug can be aerosolized and used for a chemical attack. In the early 1960s, the United States stockpiled this agent, but as it became clear that its effects would be very unpredictable, the government destroyed these reserves in the 1980s. It has been alleged (but not proved) that the Bosnian Serbs used this agent, which NATO refers to as BZ, in a chemical attack in July 1995 on civilians escaping from Srebrenica to Tuzla.

The other side of the coin is medical, therapeutic uses of atropine. Because of atropine's effect on the heart, doctors have used it for years to speed up dangerously slow heart rhythms. When patients have some kinds of heart block and other forms of slow heartbeats, intravenous atropine will often instantly and dramatically remedy the problem. Ophthalmologists occasionally use atropine drops in the eyes to intentionally dilate the pupils.

Over the years, from time to time, reports have appeared in the medical literature about cases not unlike the chemistry student that Dr. Setnik had seen. They have been infrequent, but interesting in their details.

In a striking case from 1992, a fifty-four-year-old man complained of sudden onset of blurred vision in his right eye after lifting a heavy flowerpot. On examination, his right pupil was found to be extremely dilated, but he was otherwise normal. The patient took no medications that could have this effect and had no exposure to eye drops. After taking an exhaustive history, the physicians learned that the man had been cutting a plant called angel's trumpet (*Datura suaveolens*), a member of the nightshade family and a plant known to secrete atropine. His symptoms resolved. To be 100 percent certain, one of the examining doctors obtained some of the same plant that the man had been working with. He applied a drop of the berry of the plant onto his own eye. Predictably, the doctor's pupil dilated.

In the past decade, additional reports have been published. In one Swedish article, ophthalmologists reported six separate cases of gardeners and botanists who had somehow gotten the sap from angel's trumpet into their eyes and developed dilated pupils and blurred vision. The plant is inordinately beautiful, so it is not surprising that it has become very popular in Sweden. Large delicate branches grow toward the sky and then plummet earthward. At the end of each shoot is a large white flower, about six inches long and shaped like a bell or trumpet that hangs several feet above the ground.

In a case remarkably similar to that of Shawn Matthews, doctors in San Diego reported on a twelve-year-old boy whose parents had brought him to the emergency room because of a "funny feeling" in the eye and a dilated left pupil. The remainder of his examination was normal, and he too denied having taken, touched, or been exposed to any medications or eye drops. On requestioning the boy about the details of his recent activities, the doctors found that he had been playing in his backyard that morning and had run into a plant—an angel's trumpet. The parents remembered seeing the boy playing with some of the flowers near their pond.

The same effects have been reported as a result of contact with other, related plants. Several cases of dilated pupil from the moonflower (*Datura inoxia*) have occurred. Various medications have also caused similar effects. One of the earliest published reports concerned a twenty-eight-year-old woman who consulted her optometrist after three days of having difficulty reading due to difficulty focusing her eyes. Both her pupils were large and did not constrict when light was shined in. Detailed and repeated questioning did not reveal any medication use or handling of medications. She was referred to another doctor, who got the history that the patient had been using a medicated patch to treat her motion sickness. The active ingredient in the patch was scopolamine, which is an atropine-like alkaloid that causes dilated pupils. Somehow the patient must have handled the patch, got some of the substance on her fingers, and then touched her eyes.

In 2004, a twenty-year-old woman who was being treated for leukemia complained of headache and noticed a dilated pupil on her left side. Other than that, her neurological exam was normal, but because she was being treated with strong chemotherapy agents for her cancer, she underwent a CT scan of the brain, which was normal. After this testing, the patient recalled having taken a scopolamine patch off her scalp just before the headache started.

Other cases have occurred from eye drops and from the inhaled medications that asthmatics use for treating a flare-up. In all of these cases, the nature of the problem was not revealed until the doctor eventually unearthed information that had not been offered initially.

"In medicine, we feel about 80 percent of diagnoses can usually be made by the history alone," says Setnik. "Despite all the high-technology tests we have available now, it is still the history that tells you what is wrong with somebody. If I did not have a ready explanation, I was seriously thinking about transferring him to the Boston Children's Hospital for him to have an angiogram. And so I started over again.

"Now I wanted to know if there was any possible way Shawn had gotten something into his eye. Was anyone in the family using eye drops? Was there a visitor to the house using them? Were there any old medications in the house? Then Mrs. Matthews looked up and said, 'Oh, my God! What are we putting in Fluffy's eyes?'

"'Who's Fluffy?' I asked. It turns out that Fluffy was the cat, and she had some type of eye problem that the veterinarian was treating with an ointment. Then Shawn volunteered, 'Just before I got the headache, I was sitting at my desk and Fluffy jumped up and I petted her.'

"I literally said, 'That's it!' But just to be sure, I asked Mrs. Matthews to go home and bring back Fluffy's medication. Shawn and his father stayed in the ER. About thirty minutes later, she returned and handed me a standard fifteen-gram-size aluminum tube. The label, which had been neatly typed by the vet, read '1 percent atropine ointment.'

"I told the family that Shawn's pupil would likely stay dilated for seven to ten days but that his eye would ultimately be completely normal." This case shows how powerful the drug is: Shawn hadn't put the medication in his eye. He only petted the cat, which must have gotten some of the ointment on her fur from cleaning herself. Shawn must have then rubbed his eye.

PART THREE

The Internal Milieu

~~~~~~~~~~~~~~~

On Saturday, October 5, 1985, Dr. Bernard Guyer, a pediatrician and professor at the Harvard School of Public Health, sat having lunch at an inn in New Hampshire. He felt about as relaxed as could be. He was celebrating his forty-third birthday and enjoying the crisp air at a luxurious world-class resort nestled between the White Mountains and the Connecticut River. Just after noon, along with his wife and his mother, Guyer sat down for lunch. Joining them at the table were close friends: Dr. Mary Wilson and her husband, Dr. Harvey Fineberg, and Dr. Phil Stubblefield and his wife, Linda.

In addition to it being Guyer's birthday, the group was there teaching and attending a medical conference sponsored by the School of Public Health, and the morning session had just ended. Surrounded by friends and family, Guyer was ready to enjoy a great birthday meal.

Planners of medical conferences need to find a stellar teaching faculty, but one extremely important aspect is holding them in desirable locales at the right time of year to attract as many doctors as possible to attend. Family members are welcome to come along, and between teaching sessions, break times are generally built in so that the attendees and their families can enjoy the surroundings and facilities of the chosen spot.

So for its conference on maternal and child health issues, the School of Public Health decided on a luxury resort in Whitfield, New Hampshire. The organizers chose to hold the conference in the fall, and they planned it on a weekend. Fall in New England; what could be better? If the weather would cooperate, the setting would be perfect.

And Mother Nature did not disappoint.

As the group sat in the well-appointed dining room, the afternoon conference schedule was hours away. The hotel was a classic New England resort, a large five-story wood structure. The dining room featured huge glass windows that overlooked a vast lawn set up with deck chairs and a swimming pool. The sun was still high in the mid-day sky. Almost as if it had been placed there as a prop by central casting, a large white swan had settled in the pool. Beyond the lawn lay the full panorama of a forest full of evergreens, oaks, sugar maples, aspens, beeches, and birches. The day's tempo was as slow as the metamorphosis of the surrounding trees, whose leaves were beginning to blush crimson, flash scarlet, blaze orange and yellow, against a backdrop of every shade of green imaginable.

The notion of targeting a conference in northern New England during the fall to take advantage of the foliage seems completely natural to us now, but it wasn't always that way. Over a century and a half ago, during his time at Walden Pond, Henry David Thoreau was one of the first to describe the magical quality of fall in New England. In his 1862 essay "Autumnal Tints," he wrote, "October is the month of painted leaves. Their rich glow now flashes round the world." He described purple grasses, red maples, scarlet oaks, chrome yellow poplars, and lemon yellow elms. Thoreau was ahead of his time in his appreciation of the fall foliage season. The cottage industry of tourists flocking north to enjoy and photograph the brilliant rainbow of color was not part of the collective consciousness until the last quarter of the nineteenth century.

The first European settlers cleared large tracts of land for farming and grazing animals, so there was likely less color to be appreciated. But beyond that simple fact, the color did not seem to make an impression. Despite their recording extremely detailed notes about the nature around them, the early inhabitants rarely mentioned the changes of leaf color in autumn. Even Thoreau noted that "the autumnal change of our woods has not made a deep impression on our own literature yet. October has hardly tinged our poetry." He continued: "A great many, who have spent their lives in cities, and have never chanced to come into the country at this season, have never seen this, the flower, or rather the ripe fruit, of the year. I remember riding with one such citizen, who, though a fortnight too late for the most brilliant tints, was taken by surprise, and would not believe that there had been any brighter. He had never heard of this phenomenon before."

As fertile agricultural lands were developed in the West, the amount of undeveloped land in the Northeast increased; the expanse of forest grew. Some have suggested that New Englanders began appreciating the color of their forests each fall at around the same time as the Impressionist movement in painting became the rage in Europe. And of course the automobile opened this territory up to "leaf peepers," visitors from southern New England and other more remote areas who travel to the region with the sole goal of observing the foliage. In modern times, fall in New England has become a full-fledged tourist industry.

Bernard felt lucky to be dining with family and friends in such a lovely place on his birthday. The group decided to have the inn's planned luncheon menu, which included five courses—appetizer, soup, salad, entrée, and dessert. There were choices for each of the courses, seafood, pork, vegetables, beef, chicken, and more. They tried a variety of dishes, but for the entrée, Guyer and most of the others selected the fresh bluefish seasoned with paprika. The mood was lighthearted, the pace relaxed, until halfway through coffee and dessert, when the meal came to an abrupt halt as Guyer's mother turned to her son and said, "You're all red!"

Phil Stubblefield, a gynecologist, recalls joking, "You're too young for hot flashes, Bernie. Maybe we ought to prescribe some estrogens."

The group laughed, but then the room began to feel stuffy and oppressive to him, so Guyer decided to go outside. "I felt hot," he recalls, "and a bit dizzy; I wanted fresh air. I left the dining room, and as I crossed the hotel lobby I passed by a mirror. Sure enough, my face was red as a beet! Then I went out onto the porch and tried to analyze what was happening."

The symptoms had started abruptly; he felt flushed, hot, and dizzy. His skin, especially on his face, was intensely scarlet. He checked his pulse and it was racing.

Guyer's initial self-diagnosis was an anxiety attack, but that theory suffered from one glaring and obvious problem: he wasn't feeling the least bit anxious. Everyone at the table was a close friend or family member. He was away for a fun weekend in a beautiful location. Guyer had been thoroughly enjoying himself.

Another possibility that crossed his mind was an allergic reaction, either to a food he had eaten, maybe an additive, or to something in the environment.

Allergic reactions are the body's response to a foreign protein or other substance. Special types of white blood cells recognize the outside intruder (called an antigen) and begin to release chemicals that cause the allergic reaction; the best known of these chemicals is called histamine. Histamine and other mediators of allergic reactions can lead to skin rashes, especially hives, or constriction of the upper and lower airway passages, manifesting as shortness of breath. In severe reactions, the blood pressure can plummet to dangerous levels, and in the rare case, patients can die if the reaction goes unchecked.

A few minutes later, Phil Stubblefield strolled out onto the porch to check on his friend. "Phil and I talked for a while," recalls Guyer. "Then I noticed the strangest thing. 'Phil,' I said, 'you're turning red too!'"

"That's when I began to feel it," Stubblefield recalls. "I was hot all over. I had a headache, and it was difficult to stand, I was so dizzy."

Stubblefield and Guyer went to Stubblefield's room, where, with their families clustered around, they lay on adjacent twin beds, scarlet-faced and open-collared, comparing notes. Although they were both physicians, they followed the old adage, "A doctor who treats himself has a fool for a patient," and consulted the hotel doctor. The hotel physician agreed with them that a hospital visit seemed unnecessary at the moment, as their symptoms were neither progressing nor seemed to be life threatening. At the same time, they all remained puzzled about the cause of these mysterious symptoms. An anxiety attack was now out of the question, and the likelihood that two men were both simultaneously suffering from an allergic reaction seemed remote. But if not that, what was causing this bizarre reaction?

They decided to call in Drs. Mary Wilson and Harvey Fineberg, one of the couples that had just eaten lunch with them. Wilson was the chief of infectious diseases at Mount Auburn Hospital in Cambridge, Massachusetts. As a specialist in infectious diseases, she was used to diagnosing unusual ailments and sorting through various clues to decipher which ones were germane and which could be discarded. In this case, however, she had suspected the diagnosis even before she left the lunch table. She was pretty sure that Guyer was suffering from scombroid poisoning, and she was equally certain that the bluefish was the culprit.

Scombroid poisoning is an acute illness caused by eating fish that has not been handled or refrigerated properly, which leads to contamination by bacteria and their toxic by-products. It is sometimes confused with an allergic reaction to eating fish because of the overlap of symptoms. The word itself derives both from the Greek *skombros* and the Latin *scomber*, both of which refer to a particular fish, the mackerel. In scientific terminology, the Scombridae are a family of fish that include such favorites as tuna, mackerel, albacore, bonito, and swordfish. These fish are large, pelagic (oceangoing), rapid swimming fish that have been an important source of human food for many centuries.

In spite of the name, it is not uncommon for nonscombroid fish (among them bluefish, herring, anchovies, mahi-mahi, and sardines) to also cause the exact same symptoms. Scombroid poisoning is common and occurs in both the tropics and temperate climates.

Fish and seafood are an incredibly important and usually safe food source. Like any product that originates in nature, however, there are potential risks. In 1987, for example, Americans purchased more than 3.5 billion pounds of commercially caught seafood—about fifteen pounds for every person per year. This figure does not count the two pounds per person that is recreationally caught. Not all of this food is safe, at least not by the time it reaches your dinner plate.

From 1980 to 1994, the New York State Department of Public Health documented 339 separate seafood-associated outbreaks of illness involving nearly 4,000 patients, 76 of whom were hospitalized, and 4 of whom died. During this period, seafood poisoning accounted for nearly 20 percent of all reported food-borne illnesses. Shellfish were the most frequently implicated type of seafood (two-thirds of all seafood-related outbreaks). In the cases where it was possible to pinpoint a specific cause, scombroid poisoning accounted for nearly half of them. Of the scombroid outbreaks, the most common source was tuna, followed by bluefish.

Symptoms of scombroid poisoning develop a few minutes to a few hours after eating the fish, and usually last four to six hours. Victims have one or a number of distressing symptoms: bright red flushing, especially of the upper body, itching and hives, headache, dizziness and rapid pulse, burning or blistering of the mouth, nausea, vomiting and sometimes diarrhea, abdominal cramps, and occasionally wheezing. Some patients later say that the suspect fish had a sharp peppery taste. On rare occasions, life-threatening symptoms such as severe wheezing or very low blood pressure can occur. If these symptoms seem similar to those of an allergic reaction, it is because they are both caused, at least in part, by high histamine levels in the patient's blood.

That said, if identified correctly, scombroid is easily treated with antihistamines, and the outcome is usually quite good.

For scombroid poisoning to occur, three conditions are necessary. First, the fish's meat must contain the amino acid histidine, which is found in many dark-fleshed bony fish. Second, microorganisms that produce histidine decarboxylase, an enzyme that breaks down the histidine, must be present. Such bacteria are normal residents in many fish. Third, time and temperature conditions must favor the production and accumulation of the breakdown products (histamine and others) that, when ingested by the unwary consumer, produce the symptoms. Fish kept at room temperature for as little as three to four hours can generate toxic levels of those substances, which accumulate in the flesh. To prove the diagnosis of scombroid poisoning, the fish must be tested in the laboratory for histamine and other vile-sounding chemicals, such as putrescine and cadaverine.

Part of the reason for Dr. Wilson's swift diagnosis was the fish's slightly peppery taste, which at the time of the meal she had ascribed to the paprika. Scombroid poisoning also came quickly to mind because she had been a victim of it years before, after eating bluefish in a small, popular restaurant in Cambridge when she was an infectious-diseases trainee at Harvard. She suspected it from the very beginning when Guyer began to feel ill, but when Stubblefield developed the same symptoms, it all but clinched the diagnosis.

If Wilson's on-the-spot diagnosis proved correct, and if the inn failed to remove the fish from that night's dinner menu, dozens more cases could occur; the dining room seated a couple of hundred people, and this was peak foliage season, so the place was packed. Therefore, after Stubblefield and Guyer called the hotel doctor, Fineberg telephoned the hotel manager. "I reported our concern about the bluefish and suggested it would be inadvisable to serve it for dinner," he recalls. The manager replied that he had just called an ambulance for another sick lunch patron, and agreed he would not be serving the fish. "I reassured him that if we were right, nobody would die—although they might feel like they were going to," says Fineberg.

Shortly thereafter, Wilson and Fineberg also developed facial flushing and headaches. Of the five people at the table who had eaten the bluefish, all except Guyer's mother had now fallen ill. Once the bluefish was eliminated from the menu, no new cases developed.

Some stories might have ended there. Early Monday morning, however, Wilson phoned the CDC in Atlanta seeking advice about how to further evaluate this aborted epidemic. She was put in touch with Paul Etkind, the state epidemiologist for Massachusetts, who immediately launched a two-pronged investigation. First he set out to track the path of the fish from the distributor to the lunch table. Second, he distributed questionnaires to participants at the medical conference, the responses to which ultimately confirmed the suspicion that the bluefish and no other food was the culprit. Five of the seven diners who ate the bluefish had fallen ill, but no one who had not eaten the fish got sick. The likelihood of this pattern occurring by chance was close to nil.

Because the fish had been served in New Hampshire, Etkind notified his northern counterpart, Joyce Cournoyer, who promptly dispatched a field investigator. Etkind later learned that the fish had been purchased from a large Boston distributor. A team of examiners visited the supplier, tracking each step in how the fish was handled from the fishing vessel to the trucks that delivered it to the restaurants and other buyers. They checked temperatures of storage lockers and assessed the refrigerated trucks. This thorough investigation cleared the supplier of any wrongdoing.

John Seiferth, a district sanitarian for the New Hampshire Department of Public Health, was also pressed into duty rapidly. "I was in North Conway when I received the call late Monday morning detailing the outbreak of presumed scombroid poisoning at the inn. I immediately headed north on Route 302 to inspect the premises. I recalled that I had been there just a few months before on a routine inspection."

The notes from his earlier visit, which took three hours, showed numerous lapses in sanitary protocol. The concluding paragraph of the report advised the establishment: "Keep cold foods cold and hot foods hot. The large kettle of melted butter must be refrigerated to 45 degrees or less, or heated to 140 degrees or higher. Meats and fish when in preparation are to be put back in the cooler if not being cooked. Each cooler is to have a thermometer." His report listed other issues as well, and the establishment was given just a 57 percent positive rating.

When Seiferth arrived this time, the investigation was anything but routine; a public-health nurse was already waiting for him. They met on the same porch where Guyer had stood just two days earlier, trying to analyze his symptoms.

When John Seiferth enters an establishment, he is not usually greeted like royalty. "People are not happy to see me; they are on the defensive, but they generally cooperate," he says. "I remember going into the inn and talking to the chef. I asked him if any of the bluefish from Saturday's lunch was still available. He told me that it had been thrown out yesterday and then he abruptly left the room.

"The nurse and I looked at each other. We both thought this hasty exit odd," recalls Seiferth. But they continued their orderly examination of the premises, trying to trace the travels of the bluefish.

What they determined was that the inn had ordered one hundred pounds of bluefish on September 10 from the Boston distributor, and it was delivered on September 12. The fish was then separated into four twenty-five-pound blocks, which were frozen in the inn's freezer. One of the blocks had been transferred to a walk-in refrigerator on October 1 to thaw for use on the next day. That fish was not served the next day, however, and remained in the walk-in cooler. A second twenty-five-pound block was defrosted in the cooler on October 4. The fish served to Guyer and his party came from those two blocks.

Two staff members, both cooks, said they had sampled the cooked bluefish with no ill effects. They both had an alternative theory about why some of the people got sick on that Saturday. The cooks believed that the problem was due to some residual soap on the silverware; that, they insisted, would explain why some people who ate the bluefish did not get sick.

In the cooler, Seiferth found cod and Boston scrod, Norwegian salmon and pollock, sole and blackfish, but no bluefish. He spent four hours inspecting the kitchen, recorded various temperatures, duly noted several health-code violations that he found, and then left.

On his way out, though, he still felt uneasy about the chef's awkward departure, and he thought it odd that none of the fish remained. On a hunch, Seiferth strolled around to the back of the inn, where the trash dumpsters stood. His sixth sense yielded an impressive dividend: a large amount of still-frozen bluefish in one of the dumpsters.

"The fact that the fish was still frozen was crucial for two reasons," recalls Seiferth. "First, it meant that the chef had not been forthright, because the weather had definitely been too warm for the fish to have stayed frozen overnight. And second, because the fish had not decayed, we would be able to do a meaningful chemical analysis."

The New Hampshire lab lacked the means for performing the necessary tests, so the fish was transported to the state line, where—as if it were nuclear waste or smuggled drugs—it was transferred to the custody of Massachusetts authorities, who brought it to the state laboratory facilities in Jamaica Plain. There, the bluefish was defrosted under controlled conditions and tested. Normal levels of histamine in fish are close to zero, and the FDA has established a danger, or action, level for histamine at 50 milligrams per 100 grams of fish. In the bluefish from the resort, the Massachusetts authorities found a histamine concentration five times higher than that. Their tests for cadaverine and putrescine were also positive. According to Seiferth, the specific sample that was examined was probably the remainder of the two blocks that had been served on October 5 and then, for some questionable reason, refrozen.

The fact that the frozen fish still contained toxins highlights another important point about scombroid poisoning, most graphically illustrated by the case of the nuns and the tuna.

On August 27, 1979, off the coast of New Jersey, six amateur sports fishermen caught twenty-eight yellowfin tuna, each fish weighing between forty-five and a hundred pounds. This represented an enormous catch—far more tuna than they knew what to do with. It was also far more than they had room for in the onboard icebox. So they placed the excess fish on the deck and periodically hosed it down with seawater. Once onshore, the fishermen divided their catch. One of them took his six fish and put them in his refrigerator at home, but he did not freeze them. His sister was a nun at a nearby Catholic monastery, so he took some of his fish, and some from one of the other fishermen, to the monastery, where he donated them as a gift. He did not refrigerate the fish during the transport.

Thankful for their bounty, these nuns donated one of the fish to a neighboring convent. At this second monastery, that tuna was cut into steaks and frozen for later consumption. About a month later, the nuns from this second monastery enjoyed a meal of broiled tuna. Within a few hours, twenty-three of them abruptly became ill. Their faces turned bright scarlet; they developed headaches, diarrhea, dizziness, nausea, and vomiting. Two of the older women, both in their sixties, had to be hospitalized overnight for monitoring, intravenous fluids, and treatment with antihistamines.

The nuns at the first monastery had eaten the eight tuna the fisherman gave them on five different occasions. Twice, they experienced typical symptoms of scombroid poisoning, but they had attributed this to improper cooking, not to contaminated fish. On one occasion, just before the New Jersey state health inspectors tracked the tuna backward from the second monastery to the first one, the nuns from the first monastery decided to take no chances: this time they boiled the tuna for a full hour to eliminate the cause of their prior illness. Within minutes of eating the boiled tuna, twelve of the twenty women became sick again—facial flushing, nausea, and dizziness. When the investigators tested the bit of fish that was left, they found histamine levels of 370 milligrams per 100 grams of fish. This was even higher than what was found in the New Hampshire outbreak.

The fact that the fish was still contaminated after an hour of boiling is important. Short of divine intervention, once a fish has spoiled, nothing will render it harmless: not freezing, not cooking, neither smoking nor canning. In fact, one large outbreak of scombroid poisoning was traced back to commercially canned tuna. Even vacuum packing after cooking does not prevent the disease if the histamine has already been formed. Salting may help a bit, but some bacteria are salt tolerant and can also lead to the histamine formation. Preservatives that kill bacteria will help reduce the problem, but they do not prevent it entirely.

How does fish need to be handled? Recall that the flesh of many fish contains high levels of the amino acid histidine, but that the fish do not contain free histamine. The enzymes in bacteria that often reside on the surface of and in the gut of the fish facilitate the reaction that generates histamine from histidine. This chemical reaction will occur only when the fish are stored at too high a temperature after being caught. For example, experiments show that one can store a mackerel for nearly three weeks at freezing temperature with little if any histamine formation. However, the same fish will form high levels of histamine in just five days if it is stored at 50 degrees Fahrenheit.

The period of time that the New Jersey tuna was on deck, refrigerated but not frozen, and then transported to the first monastery allowed this chemical reaction to take place. Although there are strict regulations for the commercial fishing fleet, there are no such regulations for sports fishermen, and more than 20 percent of all fish consumed in the United States is caught by recreational fishermen. Many of the fishing vessels used by these fishermen do not have adequate refrigeration capabilities to properly maintain the fish.

Scombroid-type fish have a fourteen-day shelf life at freezing if they are chilled rapidly (reducing their internal temperature to 30 degrees in less than six hours). This shelf-life is halved, however, when it's stored at 41 degrees. It is important to remember that these time and temperature measurements include the time that fish is on the boat. Fish that is kept whole takes longer to freeze than fish that is cut open and filleted on board. Even gutting the fish without cutting it into filets will help in this equation, because removing the guts reduces the available bacteria that are crucial to the spoiling process. The bottom line is that it is important to rapidly chill the fish to the desired temperature and to maintain them at that temperature. Fish will store indefinitely if promptly frozen.

But why go through the bother of diagnosing scombroid poisoning in the first place? After all, it's not fatal, and the symptoms eventually subside even without treatment.

The first reason is that some cases are quite severe. The rapid pulse rate can be dangerous for older patients or those with preexisting cardiac conditions. As well, some patients can develop severe bronchial tube constriction, seriously low blood pressure, and, very rarely, heart failure. One British woman collapsed after eating mackerel in a restaurant in Ipswich, England. In the emergency department, she had a blood pressure of 60/40, which is dangerously low. Initially she did not respond to intravenous fluids; only when an alert doctor noted the red discoloration on her neck and chest did he administer intravenous antihistamines. Shortly after the antihistamines, the rash began to dissipate and the low blood pressure quickly resolved.

In another case reported by French physicians, a healthy thirty-six-year-old woman presented herself to a Parisian emergency department twenty minutes after eating fresh cooked tuna. She had a diffuse red rash, headache, and a very rapid pulse and respiratory rate. Hours later, despite treatment, she worsened and developed severe heart failure. Her blood pressure also dropped to perilously low levels. She recovered, but only after a three-week stay in the intensive care unit, where she had to be placed on a ventilator to support her lungs and an artificial cardiac assist device to support her heart. She nearly died.

The second reason to diagnose scombroid poisoning is a pure public health issue. New cases can be prevented by discarding suspect fish, as was done in the New Hampshire outbreak. And future epidemics can be prevented by correcting the deficient storage practices that led to the outbreak in the first place. Another benefit of correct diagnosis is that affected patients will not be mistakenly labeled as being allergic to fish. Scombroid poisoning is relatively uncommon, compared to allergic reactions, and it is certainly less well known even to some doctors.

Patients who are incorrectly labeled allergic to fish will be uncertain about exactly what kinds of fish they are allergic to. Many of the species of fish that can lead to scombroid poisoning are very common and very nutritious sources of protein and omega-3 fatty acid. Avoiding eating these fish would be completely unnecessary. An incorrect diagnosis of allergy to fish would mean a lifetime of avoiding a very healthy, not to mention tasty, food.

In addition, patients treated in a hospital can avoid costly and potentially risky interventions. If a doctor misinterprets a case of scombroid poisoning as an allergic reaction, for example, one medication that might be given is adrenaline. This medicine may be entirely appropriate for patients with a severe allergic reaction, but it will do nothing to treat scombroid. Elderly patients and those with preexisting heart disease can have serious side effects (including a heart attack) when they are given adrenaline. And last, the duration of symptoms can be lessened by prompt administration of antihistamines.

The last mystery of the New Hampshire outbreak is why Bernard Guyer's mother never became ill. She had also eaten the bluefish. Several possible explanations exist. First, patients who are taking antihistamines for environmental allergies or as anti-ulcer therapy may have the ill effects of the toxins blocked by these medications. But neither Guyer nor his mother recalls her taking any such pills.

Second, it is known that the levels of histamine in any given contaminated fish are not uniform in all parts of the fish. Levels can vary more than fourfold over a distance of just an inch from one part of the fish to another, the levels being highest in portions taken from nearest the gut. That is probably why only twelve of the twenty nuns got sick too. But the likeliest explanation for Mrs. Guyer's good fortune is that the fish served for lunch that day came from two defrosted blocks of bluefish, one of which had been thawed for four days, the other for only one day. Much less toxin would have accumulated in that second block. Her portion, lucky for her, most likely came from that batch.

~~~~~~~~~~~~~~~~~~~~~~~~~~~

Linda Corsetti, a student at Bowdoin College in Brunswick, Maine, was getting ready for a semester abroad. She had so much to do that she put off the required blood tests until the week before she was supposed to leave for Rome. After all, she was in perfect health.

"I didn't think there'd be any problem," she recalls. "I went to a lab and had the blood work done. A day later they called me up and said there was a problem, probably an error in recording the results, but to be safe, they asked me to return to have the tests repeated."

Her blood was retested, but the results were the same: a low white blood cell count with an abnormally high percentage of lymphocytes. The doctor at the school wasn't sure what the significance was; in fact, nobody was. But to Linda her abnormal blood count meant one thing. "I couldn't go to Italy with the rest of the group. I was frantic," Corsetti remembers. It was January 1984.

The causes of a low white blood cell count range from trivial to life threatening. The two most common causes of a low count are drug side effects and infections. Many different medications can cause a low white blood cell count, either because they halt the production of these cells in the bone marrow or because they induce an immune-mediated destruction of them. But Linda wasn't taking any medications at all. Infections can cause a low white count. Sometimes these infections are trivial, such as those caused by common viruses. Other, more ominous infections can also lower the white blood count, such as malaria, or life-threatening bacterial sepsis. Linda, however, had no signs of infection of any kind.

There was no evidence for a hereditary cause or a large spleen, which can sometimes sequester circulating white cells. Vitamin deficiencies can also cause low counts, but Linda's diet was excellent. An autoimmune disease, such as lupus or rheumatoid arthritis, can lower the white count, but again, these diseases simply did not fit the picture of a healthy young college student with no symptoms whatsoever. The most serious possibility of all was a disease that infiltrated the bone marrow, the place in the body where blood cells are manufactured. The most serious diseases in this category are cancer and leukemia.

The other component of Linda's white blood cell abnormality was an elevated level of a specific type of white cell—the lymphocytes. Of the more common causes of elevated lymphocytes, leukemia was also on the list, as were various infections like mononucleosis, syphilis, and tuberculosis.

With no apparent cause, and with leukemia on both lists, Corsetti's father promptly made an appointment for his daughter with a hematologist in the family's hometown of Providence, Rhode Island. By the time Corsetti walked into the doctor's office in early January 1984, her classmates were going through orientation in Rome. The doctor took a history and learned that his new patient was in excellent health. To rule out the most serious diagnosis first, he decided to directly examine Corsetti's bone marrow. After she was given a local anesthetic, a hollow needle was inserted into the pelvic bone, near the small of the back, and some bone marrow was aspirated into a syringe and examined under a microscope.

A couple of days later, the results were in: Corsetti's bone marrow was normal and the hematologist had ruled out leukemia. But there was still a mystery. What was causing the low white cell count? Given the testing that the hematologist had done, the serious infections and malignancies had been excluded; most likely it was just some virus. The doctor thought it was safe for Corsetti to catch up with her schoolmates in Rome. "The doctor told me that with the low white blood count, I might be more susceptible to infections, and he was exactly right," she recalls. "The first week I was in Rome, I came down with a really bad virus and had to stay in the infirmary at the dorm for several days. I was really sick; I even thought about coming home, but I didn't want to alarm anybody. Also, by that point, I'd have missed out on Italy, missed my semester at Bowdoin, and would have had to graduate late."

So she stuck it out. Corsetti recuperated in the infirmary and went on to enjoy a glorious semester abroad in the Eternal City.

She came home in June 1984, finished her senior year at Bowdoin, and graduated in the spring of 1985. Thinking back, she says that she may have been a bit irritable at times. She may have cried more easily than normal. And she had a voracious appetite. John Carnivale, then her boyfriend and now her husband, was a football player at Bowdoin, weighing in at 215 pounds. "Linda would go fork for fork with me, and I ate a lot," he says. "And after the meal, she'd still be hungry." But she didn't gain any weight.

After graduation, Corsetti took a front-desk job at the Omni Parker House in Boston. "My hours were crazy," she says. "Sometimes I'd work till 11 PM, and then have to be back at 7 AM. My appetite was still enormous, but I began losing weight. I had no patience at all; I must have been impossible to work with. And I couldn't deal with the customers or the complaints. I threatened to quit every other day."

One very cold night in January 1986, Corsetti, Carnivale, and her family went to a play. Despite freezing temperatures, she wore only a sweater. "I remember my father yelling at me, 'You don't take care of yourself. You don't dress properly.' But I felt perfectly comfortable," recalls Corsetti.

The play was presented by the second-year class at Harvard Medical School, where her brother John was a student. That same month, he was studying endocrinology with Dr. Ron Arky, the Charles Davidson Professor of Medicine at the medical school and chief of medicine at the Mount Auburn Hospital in Cambridge. As John Corsetti listened to Arky explain various endocrine conditions, he thought that some of them sounded all too familiar; his sister's symptoms matched those of the teaching case. He recalled: "It first struck me when she was cutting my hair one day. I was taking endocrine as a second-year medical student. My apartment was very cool but Linda felt very hot. She took off her sweatshirt and was still complaining that the apartment was too hot. The next day, I spoke to Dr. Arky."

Remembers Arky: "After a lecture one day, John came up to me and asked me to see his sister as a patient. I saw her late one February afternoon, and there was no question that she had classic hyperthyroidism."

The thyroid gland straddles the windpipe just below the Adam's apple in the neck. It is a ductless gland that manufactures the hormone thyroxine, which it secretes directly into the bloodstream. The word "thyroid" comes from the Greek *threos*, for shield-shaped. Leonardo da Vinci was one of the first to identify the gland in sketches he made in 1511. The material came from anatomical studies done at the Santa Maria Nuova, a hospital that still stands not far from the Duomo in Florence.

Thyroxine controls the body's metabolic rate. Normally, the amount of the hormone circulating in the body ranges from roughly five to eleven micrograms per one hundred cubic centimeters of blood. That narrow range is maintained by intricate feedback loops controlled by the hypothalamus and the pituitary gland, the body's master regulators, deep in the brain. It is a delicate balance. Too much thyroxine, a condition known as thyrotoxicosis or hyperthyroidism, speeds up the metabolism, and too little slows it down. There are several different conditions that can lead to thyrotoxicosis. Benign and malignant tumors of the gland, if they secrete the hormone (and many do not), can result in hyperthyroidism. Sometimes a nodule or inflammation of the gland will do the same. And then there is the condition that we now call Graves' disease.

In 1835, Robert J. Graves, an Irish physician, described four patients with the disease that now bears his name. Robert James Graves was born in Dublin in 1796. He studied the classics and science as an undergraduate student, and received his medical degree at age twenty-three from Trinity College in Dublin. On graduating first in his class in 1818, he was awarded Trinity's gold medal. Like many physicians in his time, Graves served a peripatetic apprenticeship, traveling across continental Europe to study with the masters in France, Germany, and Austria. He was greatly influenced by the clinical teaching methods in Germany. Even beyond medicine, he led a fascinating life.

So well did he learn German that he was once arrested as a German spy in Austria, after having forgotten his passport. He was detained for a fortnight, as the authorities refused to believe that any Irishman could speak their language so fluently. He traveled and painted for a while in Rome and Florence with an older man he befriended. Only months later did he learn that his painting companion was J. M. W. Turner.

He returned to Dublin in 1821 and began a very successful private practice as well as taking a teaching post at the university, where he would begin his teaching rounds early in the morning, illuminated by candlelight. He brought some of the bedside teaching techniques that he had seen in Germany back to Ireland. As many as one hundred students would pack into his afternoon lectures, which were delivered with quite a bit of theatrics. He also was one of the first physicians to deliver his lectures not in Latin but in English. Of educating doctors, Graves said: "The physicians' profession is acquaintance with disease and its remedies. It is not chemistry, it is not anatomy, it is not physic, it is not physiology, it is disease." Once again taking the lead of the great teachers of medicine from the continent, Graves insisted that his students attend autopsies of their patients in order to better understand the symptoms and signs that had preceded their deaths.

Although Robert Graves is best known for his description of hyperthyroidism, his collected lectures covered the entire corpus of medicine—cardiology, chest diseases, neurology, syphilis, typhoid fever, and other common infectious diseases of his time. The description of hyperthyroidism was made by others before him. A twelfth-century Persian physician named Sayyid Ismail Al-Jurjani reported an association of goiter (a swelling of the thyroid gland) and exophthalmos (bulging eyes). The word "goiter" derives from the Latin *guttur*, meaning throat. The first known record of a goiter (but not the association with the eye findings) was by the Chinese physician Tshui Chih-Thi in 85 AD. When a goiter secretes thyroxine into the bloodstream, hyperthyroidism occurs, and exophthalmos is one symptom of hyperthyroidism.

The next person to describe hyperthyroidism was an esteemed British physician named Caleb Hillier Parry. In 1786, he described five cases of exophthalmic goiter, palpitation, and anxiety. He wrote of these patients, "the eyes were protruded from their sockets, faces exhibited an appearance of agitation and distress, the heart beat was so violent that each systole of the heart shook the whole thorax." His report, however, was not published until years after his death. In 1800, an Italian doctor, Giuseppe Flajani, also reported some cases of the same disease. In fairness, these three men had priority over Graves.

Graves, though, composed a graphic report, initially of three patients, and this is what led to his name becoming associated with the disorder. He wrote,

I have lately seen three cases of violent and long-continued palpitations in females, in each of which the same peculiarity presented itself: enlargement of the thyroid gland; the size of this gland, at all times considerably greater than natural, was subject to remarkable variations in every one of these patients. When the palpitations were violent, the gland used notably to swell and become distended, having all the appearance of being increased in size . . . [that] had attracted forcibly the attention, both of the patients and of their friends.

The enlargement of the thyroid of which I am now speaking, seems to be essentially different from goiter, in not attaining a size at all equal to that observed in the latter disease. . . . The well-known connection which exists between the uterine functions of the female and the development of the thyroid observed at puberty renders this affection worth of attention, particularly when we find it so closely related by sympathy to those palpitations of the heart which are of so frequent occurrence in hysterical and nervous females.

Graves' first three patients (and a fourth he added shortly thereafter) all had prominent bulging eyes, a rapid metabolism, and a curious swelling in the front of the neck. Goiter is a generic term used to simply describe swelling of the thyroid. In some areas of the world, where dietary iodine is lacking, endemic goiter exists. These people do not get sufficient iodine (required for making thyroxine), so their glands enlarge, sometimes to massive proportions, in an attempt to make up for the deficiency. This is called endemic goiter. These patients are not thyrotoxic, however. They have symptoms in the neck from pressure of the goiter on the windpipe, but they do not have all of the hyperthyroid symptoms that Graves described. In Graves' disease, the degree of thyroid enlargement was much less than in endemic goiter. And Graves' patients were all female. In spite of his anachronistic and incorrect association of the uterus and the thyroid, Graves did correctly make the observation that the disease is far more common in women than in men.

Graves didn't know the cause of his patients' malady; in fact, he thought it was a cardiac problem. Today we know that Graves' disease is an autoimmune problem in which the thyroid is whipped into a frenzy by antibodies that stimulate the gland. As in the famous *I Love Lucy* episode making candy on the assembly line, the thyroid cranks out more and more thyroxine—so much that the body can't handle it.

Patients with Graves' disease can have a wide range of symptoms: heat intolerance and sweating, palpitations, nervousness, insomnia, irritability, tremors, muscle weakness, weight loss despite a good appetite, diarrhea, goiter, and the characteristic exophthalmos. In addition to the high level of thyroxine in the blood, some patients have a low white blood cell count with a high percentage of lymphocytes. This is unusual as the initial finding in Graves' disease, but it did explain Linda Corsetti's blood abnormality.

"Linda had many of these symptoms," recalls Arky, "and she had been aware of a goiter since the beginning of college. I sent off the blood work, but I was pretty sure she had Graves' disease." Corsetti's initial appointment with Dr. Arky was Wednesday, February 19, 1986. Two days later, her blood work returned. Her white blood cell count was still low, with many lymphocytes, and her thyroxine level was markedly elevated at eighteen micrograms. Arky started Corsetti on a drug called propylthiouracil, or PTU, as it's commonly known. PTU decreases the thyroid's ability to produce its hormone, but it is also one of those medications that can cause a decrease in the white blood count, so Arky had to monitor Linda's blood measurements very carefully.

Her symptoms gradually faded, but although the PTU did not affect her white blood cell count, she did become aware of other issues. Over the weeks to months after starting the PTU, she felt much better, and many of her original problems resolved. "But I started having other symptoms," she recalls. "My hair was falling out in clumps. I went sailing one day and the whole boat was covered with my hair. And on top of all that, my eyes were asymmetric and I was concerned that would be permanent."

Although her bulging eyes were clearly improving, they weren't improving at the same rate: the left eye was noticeably worse than the right one. In retrospect, the eye findings had been present for a while, but because the problem had developed slowly, she hadn't noticed it. Over the spring, summer, and fall of 1986, her symptoms of hyperthyroidism resolved, her weight normalized, and her blood work showed normal thyroid function. Although the exophthalmos was slow to resolve, she felt well. On Christmas Day, John proposed to her, and they became engaged to be married.

As is customary, a year after Arky started Corsetti on PTU, he took her off it. In 30 percent of patients with Graves' disease, the disorder goes into complete remission even after the medication is withdrawn. But not Linda Corsetti. By May, a month before her wedding, she was clearly hyperthyroid again, and in June, Arky took another blood sample to recheck her thyroxine, and this time it was twenty-four micrograms. He wrote another prescription for PTU.

Linda had other concerns. First there were the usual stresses and then some: planning a wedding and a honeymoon, looking for a house, buying a new car, and traveling back and forth between Boston and Providence. Second, she didn't want to be a bride with asymmetrical eyes.

But the major issue was the dress.

"I had gained back the fifteen pounds I had lost," she remembers, "and probably twenty more. After the engagement, I began dieting. From Christmas to May, I lost forty-five pounds. I bought a really fitted dress, and they had to keep taking it in every few weeks. I knew that if I went back on the PTU, I'd gain the weight back and never fit into the gown."

Although her untreated hyperthyroidism provided what she considered a sartorial benefit, it did create other problems. Her husband recalls, "The time around the wedding was crazy; it was hell. After one fight we nearly canceled it. Then we went to Bermuda on our honeymoon. It was hot, and Linda couldn't stand the heat. Our hotel, Grotto Bay, offered cave swimming every day between noon and 1 PM. The water was about forty-five degrees, and nobody went in—except Linda. She was there every day. Once I jumped in and I thought I'd have a heart attack."

Corsetti remembers, "Needless to say, my engagement and honeymoon were tense. I had no patience at all. Bermuda was really hot, in the nineties, and I felt like I couldn't breathe. I felt hot all the time. The only refreshing thing was this ice-cold natural pool. I'd swim in it once or twice per day. Everybody else would be saying, 'Oh my God, there's a girl swimming in the freezing water! Can you believe it?'"

Hyperthyroidism can produce all sorts of mental symptoms, from mild irritability to frank psychosis. And patients with hyperthyroidism can do odd things. Says Arky, "I've seen couples split up over hyperthyroidism. The patient will want to open all the windows in the house and the spouse will be freezing.

"The most bizarre one I'd ever had was a former secretary of mine with classical Graves' disease; she had both a goiter and the exophthalmos. She was a Jehovah's Witness and refused to have any blood drawn. We could follow very easily when her condition was exacerbated and when she had remissions merely by the heat setting in the office. Also, when she was toxic, she'd consume eight thousand calories a day without gaining weight. And she was the fastest typist that existed. She peddled the Watchtower on weekends. She would start on the corner of Longwood Avenue and Huntington Street and literally walk out Route 9 to Route 128, about ten miles and back. And she wasn't fazed by it.

"There was never any question as to when she was thyrotoxic. Her energy was unbounding and she was impossible to get along with. She worked for me for three years; finally she allowed us to draw her blood; her thyroxine was twenty-four, but she would never accept any therapy. She went elsewhere to work and I lost track of her, but she was a character of the first class—but only when she was toxic."

When Linda Corsetti Carnivale returned to Boston from Bermuda, she went back on PTU and, predictably, her symptoms cleared up. It was now clear that she was going to require definitive treatment for her Graves' disease. There are two time-honored possibilities: radioactive iodine and surgery. Arky discussed the options with his patient and her husband. Older patients generally choose the radioactive iodine; former first lady Barbara Bush selected this option for her Graves' disease. The treatment is also used in younger patients, but because of the radioactivity, some women in their childbearing years opt for surgery. The surgery —a thyroidectomy—can be tricky. Aside from the possibility of infection, heavy bleeding and damage to the adjacent parathyroid glands, accidental damage to the nerves of the larynx can lead to permanent hoarseness.

Then something happened to Linda Carnivale that forced the issue: she became pregnant. Administering PTU late in a pregnancy is dangerous, because the drug crosses the placenta and can make the baby hypothyroid, and radioactive iodine was now out of the question. So early in her second trimester, thyroid surgery was scheduled.

The evolution of thyroid surgery is one of the more colorful chapters in the history of medicine, and some of its pioneers are giants of modern surgery—Theodor Billroth, Theodor Kocher, Charles Mayo, and William Halsted. Even aside from the generic problems of adequate anesthesia and postoperative infection that confronted surgeons during the second half of the nineteenth century and the first half of the twentieth, there were other issues that were specific to thyroid surgery.

In 952 AD, a Moorish physician, Khalaf Egn Abbas, reportedly performed a successful operation to remove a goiter. He apparently used opium for sedation and hot cautery irons to stanch the bleeding. In 1791, the French surgeon Pierre-Joseph Desault operated on a twenty-eight-year-old woman with a goiter. She recovered. Despite these scattered successes, however, most surgeons avoided the procedure altogether. In 1846, Robert Liston, one of England's most audacious and skilled surgeons, said, "You could not cut the thyroid gland out of a living body in its sound condition without risking the death of the patient from hemorrhage; [thyroid surgery is] a proceeding by no means to be thought of."

The thyroid is a very vascular gland, with major arteries running in every direction, and bleeding during the operation was a major problem. Twenty years later, the Philadelphia surgeon Samuel Gross summed up this concern when he wrote: "Can the thyroid in the state of enlargement be removed? Should the surgeon be so foolhardy to undertake it . . . every stroke of the knife will be followed by a torrent of blood and lucky it would be for him if his victim lived long enough for him to finish his horrid butchery. No honest and sensible surgeon would ever engage it."

In his treatise on the subject of thyroid surgery, William Halsted, chief surgeon at the newly formed Johns Hopkins Hospital, wrote that mortality from thyroidectomy before 1850 was 40 percent. But during the second half of the nineteenth century, doctors gradually overcame the problems of anesthesia, sterile technique, and infection. European surgeons began using small metal clamps to stop intraoperative bleeding. The ability to operate in a bloodless field on an anesthetized patient, who had a good chance of not dying from a postoperative infection, set the stage for more intricate operations.

In 1860, at the age of thirty-one, Theodor Billroth became the chair of surgery at Vienna. Previously he had worked in Zurich. One of the areas in which goiter is endemic due to low dietary iodine is the region that encompasses southeastern France, northern Italy, and parts of Switzerland. This provided surgeons in this area with a steady supply of patients with large goiters (but who were not thyrotoxic). It was here that Billroth began his work in the field. Of his first thirty-six procedures (done without sterile technique), sixteen died. This dismal 36 percent mortality rate led him to abandon the procedure until the late 1870s. Then, using the sterile techniques that had since become standard, between 1877 and 1881 he did forty-eight thyroidectomies with a mortality rate of just over 8 percent.

It was Billroth's pupil, Theodor Kocher, who was a professor of surgery at Bern, who took thyroid surgery to the next level. Because Bern is part of the area of endemic goiter, Kocher rapidly gained experience in the field. During his first ten years in his post at Bern, he removed 101 goiters with only 13 deaths. Kocher became so renowned that he received the Nobel Prize in Medicine for "his work in physiology, pathology, and surgery on the thyroid gland" in 1909, the first surgeon ever to be so honored.

In 1917, weeks before he died, he presented his lifelong experience with benign goiter; in approximately five thousand cases, his mortality rate was less than 1 percent. Part of the large reduction in mortality rates had to do with general improvements in surgical procedures, including anesthesia, clamps to prevent bleeding, and sterile technique, and part was a result of the accumulated experience of surgeons.

Just as Graves had done, Halsted made his medical pilgrimage to Europe in 1878. He spent two years at the great European surgical centers, observing and learning from both Kocher and Billroth. He brought the techniques he acquired back to America and became an authority on thyroid surgery.

Mortality, however, is just one measure of the success (or failure) of a surgical procedure. Other complications must also be considered. In the case of thyroid surgery, there are several important ones. The first complication was causing the patient to become hypothyroid—too little thyroid. Kocher was the first to recognize this problem. On January 8, 1874, he performed a total thyroidectomy on an eleven-year-old girl named Marie Richsel. Kocher later reported that the referring physician contacted him to report that "the girl had become quite cretinoid. This seemed so important to me that I made every effort to examine the girl, which was not easy since this physician had died very shortly after making his report. We were all the more intent upon it since our colleague, Reverdin of Geneva, had informed us that he had observed two patients who had suffered diminution of mental capacity following goiter operations. I was highly astonished at the striking appearance of my patient. . . . She had an ugly, almost idiotic appearance. As soon as this was determined, I immediately requested all of my goiter patients to return for examination."

Of thirty-four such patients, Kocher could locate only eighteen; of those, sixteen had developed hypothyroidism. So Kocher changed his standard operation to leave a little bit of thyroid tissue behind to prevent this complication. This was before the days when thyroid extract could simply be given to treat this possible complication of thyroidectomy.

There were other pitfalls too, however. Some patients would develop tetany after thyroid surgery. Tetany, after the Greek *tetanus*, which means painful contracture, developed shortly after thyroid surgery in a variable percentage of patients. Sometimes it was transient; other cases were permanent. Patients with tetany had painful muscle spasms, especially in the hands and feet, very twitchy reflexes, and odd sensations in the body. In severe cases spasm of the larynx could result. Over time, the surgeons learned that this was due to the inadvertent removal of the tiny parathyroid glands, four glands the size of watermelon seeds that are responsible for calcium metabolism and are located on the rear surface of the thyroid. The frequency of this complication was a function of how meticulous the surgeon's technique was.

Last, nerves to the larynx lie in close proximity to the thyroid gland. If a surgeon inadvertently cut the recurrent laryngeal nerve during the operation, permanent hoarseness would result. Again, once this anatomic detail was clarified, surgeons developed techniques to avoid it.

By 1900, Europeans were light years ahead of the Americans in thyroid surgery. Halsted could find reports of only 45 operations in America up to the year 1883; by that same date, Billroth had performed 125 by himself. The metal clamps that the Europeans were using were nearly nonexistent in the United States and late to be adopted. Halsted wrote: "Few hospitals in New York, at least, possessed as many as six artery clamps in 1880. I recall vividly an operation performed by Mikulicz in 1879 in Billroth's clinic. Americans, newly arrived in Austria, we were greatly amused at seeing perhaps a dozen clamps left hanging in a wound of the neck while the operator proceeded with his dissection, and were inclined to ridicule the method as being untidy or uncouth. Slowly it dawned upon us that we in America were the novices in the art as well as the science of surgery. The value of artery clamps is not likely to be over estimated. They determine methods and effect results impossible without them. They tranquilize the operator. In a wound that is perfectly dry, and in tissues never permitted to become even stained by blood, the operator, unperturbed, may work for hours without fatigue."

The Americans caught up rapidly, though. Halsted, who performed only six cases in the first ten years that he was at Hopkins, did ninety in the next ten years (with a mortality rate of 2 percent), and by 1914, he reported on over five hundred cases of thyroidectomy in Graves' disease alone. Others, such as Charles Mayo, George Crile, and Frank Lahey, followed. By the time Lahey died in 1953, he had personally performed nearly ten thousand thyroidectomies.

Most surgeons in the United States had only a tiny fraction of that experience, however. Today, the recommendation for patients needing thyroid surgery is to have it done by a surgeon who performs at least fifty procedures per year, which is ten times more than what most American surgeons in general practice do. Linda was a sophisticated patient, and her fears were not totally unjustified. And on top of everything else, she was pregnant. Ironically, her mother also had needed thyroid surgery for Graves' disease during one of her pregnancies. Dr. Arky consulted with an experienced neck surgeon, who performed the procedure on October 10, 1988.

"Linda was hysterically afraid," recalls her husband, "and I was a wreck. The morning of surgery, I got to the hospital at four-thirty in the morning so I could be with her before they took her to the operating room at six. We knew that there was risk to the baby and to Linda." The surgery was successful, and about six months later, the Carnivales had a healthy baby boy.

Since her surgery, Linda Carnivale has felt fine. Her husband remarks on the patience she has with their son and thinks how different it all would have been if the hyperthyroidism hadn't been diagnosed and treated. "We went back to Grotto Bay last summer," he says, "and it was just as hot as during out honeymoon. Linda couldn't believe how cold the water was. Of course, it was the same temperature as before, but she couldn't stand it this time."

~~~~~~~~~

By midmorning on Tuesday, December 13, 1988, Henry Schachte of Weston, Connecticut, knew something was dreadfully wrong. That was when the abdominal pain began. "It felt like my stomach was being inflated with air," recalls the seventy-six-year-old retired advertising executive. As the day wore on, the pain intensified, and by 9 PM, Schachte knew he needed help. He threw on some pajamas and drove himself to Norwalk Hospital.

There, in the emergency department, Schachte was examined by Dr. Edward Tracey, the surgeon who had operated on him for diverticulitis eight years earlier, removing part of his colon. He had mild high blood pressure and was on a medication for that. He had had knee surgery in 1980, and some minor prostate issues. A widower for three years, Schachte lived alone and cooked for himself. He ate prudently and had recently increased his fiber consumption to lower his cholesterol. Overall, Schachte was in pretty good health for a man his age.

In the emergency department, Dr. Tracey did not like what he saw. Schachte was in moderate distress from the pain. His blood pressure was elevated. Most important, his abdomen was distended and diffusely tender. When the surgeon pressed on it, there was an involuntary tensing of the abdominal wall muscles, which is often a harbinger of serious mischief in the belly.

In an era before the routine availability of CT scans, Dr. Tracey ordered a series of plain x-rays of the abdomen. These films revealed dilated loops of small bowel, confirming the surgeon's initial diagnostic impression: Schachte had an obstruction in his small intestine.

The human intestine is a long, hollow tube that begins at the stomach and ends at the anus. It consists of two basic parts: the small intestine and the large intestine. In the stomach, various acids, enzymes, and, to some extent, mechanical motion begin the first steps of digestion of the food that is swallowed. Once the material finds its way into the first part of the intestines (called the duodenum), the principal task is to further break down the food into its basic elements and complete the process of digestion, absorbing what is useful and eliminating what is not. The three portions of the small intestine are the duodenum, which empties into the jejunum, which in turn becomes the ileum. The ileum empties into the large intestine, or colon, at the point where the appendix lies. The small intestine gets its name not from its length (it is much longer than the large intestine) but from its smaller diameter.

Although most nutrients (protein, fats, and carbohydrates) are absorbed in the small intestine, its contents remain uniformly liquid from start to finish. It is in the large intestine that water is absorbed and the waste product, stool, assumes a solid consistency.

Because it is narrow, the small intestine can become obstructed relatively easily, making such blockages a common cause for admission to a surgical ward. In patients with small bowel obstructions, the portion of the intestine proximal to the obstruction swells. As the swelling increases, the blood supply to that part of the gut is compromised, and if the obstruction is not relieved, that part of the bowel will die. This leads to perforation and infection of the abdominal cavity, or peritoneal cavity, as doctors call it. This inflammation or infection of the peritoneum is called peritonitis. The inflammation leads to fluid being drawn out of the blood vessels and accumulating in the peritoneal cavity; this in turn can cause the blood pressure to fall. Unchecked and untreated, a bowel obstruction usually results in death.

Diagnosing the presence of a bowel obstruction is the first step. The next step, finding out its cause, is also important. Although there are dozens of potential causes, most result from one of two problems—hernias and adhesions resulting from prior surgery. Sometimes, a hernia of a portion of the bowel causes a kink that blocks the flow of intestinal material. An adhesion is an area of scarring in the peritoneal cavity that also causes a loop of bowel to twist or kink, resulting in a bowel obstruction. Fifty years ago, hernias were the most common cause of obstructions, but over the past several decades, adhesions have caught up and surpassed them in frequency. Most abdominal adhesions, by far, are the result of prior abdominal surgery. Sometimes the bowel obstruction from an adhesion will fix itself; however, surgery is often necessary.

After the patient is put to sleep by an anesthesiologist, the surgeon makes an incision into the abdomen, and then "runs" the bowel, meaning that he will inspect the bowel from the duodenum to the anus, to find any pathology. Often there is a clear-cut transition point at the site of the obstruction. The surgeon snips or otherwise releases the adhesion or reduces an internal hernia, the bowel floats back to a normal position, and the surgeon closes the incision. If all goes well, it is a fairly quick and routine operation.

"I remember distinctly telling Mr. Schachte that we'd be in and out of the operating room in about an hour," says Tracey. "I should have known better. When we opened him up, it was a real mess. There were massive adhesions from the old surgery."

His dictated postoperative report spells out the details:

> On entering the peritoneum, [we found] totally fixed adhesions of the bowel to the omentum [fatty tissue that lies within the abdomen] and to the overlying peritoneum, from the diaphragm right down to the pelvis. The most proximal end and the distal ileum were of normal caliber. By tedious blunt and sharp dissection, the small bowel loops were carefully separated from one another in two areas where the bowel was fixed.
>
> After about three hours, the bowel was finally cleared and there was no one area that could be seen as the site of his obstruction. The middle aspect of the small bowel was packed with a very thick material that may have been the causative factor. This was some type of undigested vegetable material.

Dr. Tracey recalls, "We made an incision in the suspicious area of bowel. That's when this paste, the consistency of toothpaste, came out; it was totally obstructing the segment of small intestine. We filled a small bucket with the stuff." Tracey removed a two-foot-long concretion of the thick impacted goo, the consistency of soft concrete that hasn't set. He sent the material to the pathologist, but he was already pretty sure he knew what the problem was—a bezoar.

Bezoars are solid clumps of ingested material found in the alimentary canal of animals, mostly ruminants. Ruminants include cows, goats, sheep, deer, and antelopes—animals that have special four-chambered stomachs that are designed to digest their food in two steps. First they eat their food. The food sits for a while in the first two chambers; eventually, the animal regurgitates the semi-digested food, known as cud, and then begins to chew the cud. This process is called ruminating (which accounts for the use of the word "ruminate" to mean taking a long time to think about something). Occasionally, partially digested foodstuff in the stomachs of these animals begins to form. They become firm concretions, which sometimes form a solid mass as hard as a rock.

Although it may seem somewhat fantastic today, bezoars have been prized by humans for at least three millennia. The original bezoars are thought to have come from goats in the mountains of western Persia. The word "bezoar" probably derives from a combination of two old Persian words, *pâd*, meaning protector, and *zahr*, meaning poison. The combination, *pâdzahr*, is the likely the root for the Arabic *badzehr* and the Turkish *panzehir*. All of these words mean the same thing—protector from poison, or, in modern parlance, an antidote.

Consistent with this meaning, bezoars were thought to possess curative powers in times past. Bezoars taken from goats, sheep, gazelles, and probably other animals were collected and preserved to be used as medical "charms" since at least 1000 BC. Galen, a Greek physician who practiced in Rome in the second century AD and wrote extensively, had an enormous influence on medical practice well into the Renaissance. According to an article in the *British Journal of Homeopathy* written in 1841, Galen prescribed a bezoar stone in cases of jaundice and apparently was most fond of bezoars made from the stags of "eastern countries."

In the eleventh century, bezoars were introduced to Europe from the Middle East. The Europeans considered bezoars to be of enormous value. They were used to treat snake bites, plagues, and all other sorts of "evil spirits." Physicians even debated various dosages; twelve grains were used for a bite, while a weak heart or loss of sexual power was treated with only a single grain. In the late sixteenth century, the French surgeon Ambrose Paré, court physician to several kings of France and considered by some to be the father of modern surgery, was one of the most celebrated doctors in the world. He is best known today for his discoveries in the treatment of battlefield wounds. He found that a mixture of egg yolk, oil of roses, and turpentine worked better (and was immensely less painful) than the standard practice of his time, which was cauterizing the wound with boiling oil. He is less well known for an experiment he performed to test the effectiveness of treatment with bezoars.

Looking for an opportunity to see just how good a bezoar was at protecting a person from poison, Paré devised an experiment that was both simple and elegant. It may sound cruel to the modern ear, but he was using the scientific method to test a treatment that was very well accepted at the time. In 1575, a cook in the imperial court's household had stolen some fine silverware. The cook agreed to be poisoned rather than hanged. Paré decided that he would administer a bezoar to see if it saved the man.

The cook was given the poison, and then the bezoar. According to Paré: "An hour after [he took the poison], I found him on the ground on his hands and feet like an animal with his tongue hanging out of his mouth, his eyes wild, vomiting, with blood pouring from his ears, nose, and mouth. Eventually he died in great torment, seven hours after I gave him the poison. I opened his body and found the bottom of the stomach dry, as if it had been burned." The king commanded that the useless bezoar be destroyed.

Even after Paré's experiment, bezoars continued to be valued for their curative powers. One famous claim in British case law, *Chandelor v. Lopus* in 1603, first introduced the notion of caveat emptor, or "buyer beware." The dispute in the case had to do with the alleged fraudulent sale and purchase of a bezoar. When the Spanish began to colonize the New World, they were sending back numerous ships laden with treasure—silver, gold, emeralds, and other precious gems. In early September 1622, the galleon *Nuestra Señora de Atocha* and a fleet of other ships, filled with riches that would finance Spain's participation in the Thirty Years' War, set off from Havana. The ships were quickly caught in the first hurricane of the season, just east of Key West, Florida. Most of the flotilla escaped, but the *Atocha* and two other ships quickly sank. Only 5 of the 265 passengers and crew members survived. The fortune they carried lay lost at the bottom of the Caribbean until 1985, when some

American treasure hunters finally located the wreck. Among the salvaged hoard, worth hundreds of millions of dollars, were silver bars and coins, gold bars, and enormous emeralds. So valuable were bezoars to the seventeenth-century Spaniards that ten of them (most likely of llama or alpaca origin) were stored in a silver case to be transported back to Madrid.

In the outbreak of bubonic plague that hit London in 1665, bezoars were still being used. However, some prominent physicians of the day were skeptical. One, Nathaniel Hodges, wrote in 1672, "For Ages together, the Oriental Bezoar still hath so great a name; yet without having an Inclination to contradict a received Opinion, I have been so convinced by a Multitude of Trials, that the Truth will speak for itself, which manifestly denies its Virtues to be at all equivalent to its value. And I have given it in Powder many times to 40 or 50 Grains, without any manner of Effect. And I dare affirm that the Bezoar with which I made these trials was genuine."

In more modern times, as recently as 1962, a gold-framed bezoar was included in Queen Elizabeth's crown jewels. Bezoars have even made their way into popular fiction. In the first Harry Potter book, during his Potions lessons, Harry is introduced to the bezoar. Later, in the Goblet of Fire, Harry forgets to add the bezoar to an antidote he is preparing. In yet another episode, when his best friend Ron is poisoned, Harry saves his life by administering a bezoar. Both in medicine and fiction, bezoars have played a long and colorful role in human history.

What Dr. Tracey was concerned about was not some magical potion derived from the ruminant stomach of a Persian antelope but a serious condition that could be at the root of his patient's abdominal symptoms. Medically, a bezoar in human beings is the same kind of concretion of foreign material that develops in animals. But in humans, bezoars can accumulate to a size that obstructs the bowel or stomach. Bezoars are formed when hairs (trichobezoars) or vegetable fibers (phytobezoars) are ingested but not digested. Bezoars usually develop in the stomach and remain there, where they can cause pain, weight loss, and diminished appetite, sometimes mimicking a cancer. Often, they form in people with abnormal gastric function due to ulcer surgery or diabetes. Occasionally the material can make its way into the small or large intestine, where it plugs up the works. Bezoars are more common in children because they have smaller intestines.

There is a long list of foods that have been reported to cause bezoars. In some areas of the world where the persimmon is a popular fruit, it is also the commonest cause of bezoars. An eleven-year-old child from Cincinnati who had had prior abdominal surgery developed a bowel obstruction from eating a large amount of peanuts and peanut butter. In a two-year-old, the obstruction was caused by a large wad of chewing gum that obstructed the distal colon. Popcorn, sunflower seeds, oranges, mushrooms, and other high fiber foods have also been implicated. In one large series of cases, patients who were toothless seemed to have a higher incidence of bezoars.

Recently, in a strange twist on the notion of side effects, medicines have been reported to cause bezoars; these are called pharmacobezoars. One is the psyllium husk, which is used to treat constipation; a twenty-three-year-old woman developed a colonic obstruction from eating too much psyllium. Cholestyramine is a medication used to lower serum cholesterol and to treat certain liver diseases. In one unfortunate toddler with a congenital bile duct disease, cholestyramine was prescribed and resulted in colonic bezoar that required surgical treatment.

An experienced surgeon, Tracey had seen his share of bezoars, and he once cared for a patient whose small intestine had become packed with mushroom particles. "The guy worked in a pizza parlor," says Tracey, "and he used to eat all the mushrooms used on the pizzas." But Schachte wasn't on any exotic diet—or was he?

Like millions of Americans, Henry Schachte had been concerned about his cholesterol level. Cholesterol is a natural substance manufactured in the liver and is a necessary building block for all human cells. During the 1980s, the National Institutes of Health began an all-out campaign to raise Americans' consciousness about cholesterol. There was a great debate in the medical and lay literature about how important cholesterol reduction is and by what means it should be accomplished, but there was consensus that high serum cholesterol levels are associated with an elevated risk of coronary heart disease, America's number one killer.

One by-product of cholesterol's new notoriety is that it is nearly impossible to steer through a food market without being assaulted by signs extolling the virtues of fiber. Most people now understand that greater consumption of dietary fiber may be related to lower cholesterol levels; consequently, we have become a society obsessed by dietary fiber. In part, this obsession resulted from the findings of a British researcher working in Africa in the 1970s, Denis Burkitt, and his colleague Hugh Trowell, who found that many of the diseases common in developed countries such as diabetes, hypertension, coronary artery disease, and diverticulosis were far less common in Africa. They connected the difference to the amount of fiber in the diet.

Burkitt studied the bowel movements of indigenous Africans and British people. He found that the Africans passed more than twice (and as much as four times) the bulk of stool as sailors in the Royal Navy. He and his co-workers hypothesized that the higher consumption of fiber in the African diet resulted in a greater amount of stool and decreased transit time in the colon. When he lectured, Burkitt would often punctuate his slide presentation with photographs of human feces that he took during his morning walks in the African bush. An Irishman, he was blunt and said, to paraphrase, that "the health of a country's people could be determined by the size of their stools and whether they floated or sank, not by their technology."

Burkitt wrote, "It is now generally accepted that the major factor causative of diverticular disease is a deficiency of fibre in the diet, and my colleagues and I have argued that this may also contribute to the causation of appendicitis. Both diseases are related to the consistency and volume of intestinal content, both of which are governed by the fibre content of the diet. Bowel behaviour was examined in communities with low, high, and intermediate frequency of colorectal cancer, and it was found that where faecal output was 300–500 g/day and mouth to anus transit times around 30 hours, cancer and its associated diseases were rare, but where, as in North America and Western Europe, output was only 80–120 g/day, and transit times exceeded three days, these illnesses were common."

Burkitt lectured in Britain and the United States, preaching the virtues of a natural diet rich in unprocessed foods and natural fiber and decrying the typical Western diet of white flour and highly refined sugars. Numerous scientific studies showed the benefits of a high fiber diet. The incidence of diabetes was lower. Cholesterol levels fell. Diverticulosis of the large intestine, a serious problem in which small outpouchings on the colon can became obstructed, inflamed, and infected, was less common. More minor but common health issues, such as constipation and hemorrhoids, were shown to be less widespread.

This issue became so pervasive that *Time* magazine covered the story in 1974. The following year, Burkitt and Trowell wrote a book about fiber. The foreword of their book says: "Once every 10 years or so a new idea emerges about the cause of disease that captures the imagination and, for a time, seems to provide a key to the understanding of many of these diseases whose aetiology was previously unknown. . . . To these we may now add a deficiency of dietary fiber. But whether it will be as seminal an idea as that of vitamin deficiency we shall probably not know for another 10 years." Some of Burkitt's ideas have not withstood the test of time (the relationship between low fiber and colon cancer has been questioned in more recent studies), but his basic theories and findings about a high fiber diet and health have had a sustaining influence.

It is also clear now that not all fibers are created equal. According to the American Dietetic Association, "dietary fiber is primarily the storage and cell wall polysaccharides of plants that cannot be hydrolyzed by human digestive enzymes." There are two types of fiber—soluble and insoluble. And the two types have different effects on cholesterol levels.

Dr. Don Levy is an internist who practices in Cambridge, Massachusetts. He specializes in lipid disorders and is an instructor at Harvard Medical School. Says Levy, "If you took insoluble fiber, like wheat bran, and put it into a glass of water, it would just sit at the bottom and not absorb any water. Soluble fiber, on the other hand, would absorb water and form a gooey, viscous gel." Only soluble fibers, such as oat bran and beans, can lower serum cholesterol levels.

No one understands how it works yet. Dr. James Anderson, a veteran researcher on the effects of soluble fiber, suggests that oat bran leaches cholesterol out of the system by causing bile acids (cholesterol by-products made in the liver and circulated in the intestine) to be eliminated in the gut. Additionally, when oat bran reaches the large intestine, it undergoes fermentation, releasing chemicals called fatty acids, which decrease cholesterol production. So less is made and more is lost, resulting in less cholesterol in the system. And there seems to be a selective decrease in low-density lipoproteins (LDL), commonly known as "the bad cholesterol" because they are usually associated with atherosclerosis, or hardening of the arteries. It's also possible, of course, that the more bran and fiber one eats, the more full one feels, and therefore the less fatty and other unhealthy foods one eats.

All of this meant that by the 1980s, everybody was talking about fiber, and oat bran was one of the darlings of the fiber world. It was everywhere, even in bookstores. One book published in 1987, *The Eight-Week Cholesterol Cure* by Robert E. Kowalski, makes a persuasive argument for eating oat bran. At the end of his book, Kowalski included many recipes for cooking with oat bran, but the cornerstone of his diet was the oat bran muffin.

The book certainly persuaded Henry Schachte. His daughter recalls, "The idea about the oat bran came from my brother, who had had a heart attack and had cholesterol problems. I think he told dad about the book. Dad bought a copy and I remember him thinking 'this is it.' This would cure all his problems. He wasn't abusive about it but he thought it was a great thing. He was going to make his own muffins. I remember him saying all the local health food stores were out of oat flour."

The recipe in the book calls for fairly standard ingredients—milk, egg, sweetener, baking powder—and two and a half cups of oat bran to make twelve muffins. Shortly after Schachte read the muffin recipe, he found a store where he could buy the oat bran, and he set about baking muffins. From December 3 to December 13, he ate about four muffins a day (Kowalski recommends three). Little did Schachte know that, over the course of those ten days, he was slowly stuffing his small intestine full of the partially digested muffins.

Schachte wasn't the first human in history to develop a bowel obstruction from fiber. A thirty-four-year-old was instructed by his physician to eat a large bowl of bran cereal each morning to treat his chronic constipation. Ten days after starting this new regimen, he developed abdominal pain, vomiting, and fever. As in Schachte's case, the belly was tender, and x-rays showed loops of swollen intestine. At surgery, there was no hernia and no adhesions, but a stretch of the mid-ileum a foot and a half long was filled with a pasty mass that was too thick to simply be pushed from the outside with the surgeon's fingers into the colon. That surgeon also needed to cut into the bowel and remove the material, which turned out on pathological examination to be "plant fiber." A young man without any previous surgery, the patient went on to have an uneventful postoperative course.

Still, high fiber diets are very safe according to Dr. Levy. Certain precautions should be taken. Any new dietary routine can lead to changes in a person's digestion. Because fiber passes through the gut unchanged, then undergoes fermentation in the colon, it produces gas. This can cause cramps and bloating as well as some socially unpleasant side effects.

"It's important to begin slowly," says Levy, "and to gradually build up the amount of dietary fiber. This may take a period of several weeks. And it's also very important to increase the amounts of fluids, because the soluble fibers will absorb lots of water in the intestine." This may be especially important for someone who has had abdominal surgery or has abnormal bowel function, although Tracey knows of another case of an obstruction caused by oat bran in a person who had never had prior surgery.

The pathologist's examination of the contents of Schachte's intestine verified Tracey's diagnosis: it was a phytobezoar composed of oat bran. Despite this incident, bezoars from oat bran must be very unusual, given the number of people eating oat bran in this country and the rarity of that complication. To put it all in perspective, Levy points out that "much of the world regularly eats far more fiber than we do without ill effects."

Schachte's post-op recovery was long and rocky. He awakened from surgery with a tube coming out of his nose to help decompress his stomach, and another coming directly out of his abdomen that Tracey had placed as a drain in case of infection inside the abdomen. His daughter remembers a call from Dr. Tracey the morning after surgery. "His expression was something like, 'he was stuffed like a turkey.' Dad went through an incredibly rough time afterward." Tracey's discharge summary noted that "his postoperative period was complicated by very slow return of bowel function probably due to his severe and extensive adhesions." He also developed another bout of pain from a small bowel adhesion, but fortunately Tracey was able to pull him through this episode without another surgery. Schachte himself recalls needing large doses of pain medicines that gave him very vivid and very bad dreams.

Finally, after three weeks in the hospital, he was well enough to be discharged. He remembers being "alarmed that the author was not a doctor, just a medical writer. I felt a bit tricked and angry." When asked about advice for others who are contemplating starting a high fiber diet, he said, "if you ever had anything that could leave scar tissue in the abdomen, certainly check with your doctor first."

Ultimately he recovered completely and is well again, but he avoids oat bran like the plague.

~~~~~~~~~~~~~~~~~~~~~~~~

Joanne Young was the kind of person who didn't just worry about her health; she did something about it. In fact, the forty-eight-year-old Massachusetts woman had taken exceptionally good care of herself for years, jogging five miles daily, eating a nutritious diet, abstaining from smoking, and limiting her alcohol intake to rare social occasions.

So when her feet became swollen during a vacation to Hawaii in April 1981, she dismissed it as nothing more than simple water retention. "I figured it was due to the flying or whatever, but after I returned home, my legs were still quite swollen and all the extra pounds seemed to be concentrated in my middle. I felt all right though, so I kept up my running. At one point I remember figuring, 'Oh well, this is the beginning of menopause,'" Ms. Young recalls. By late May however, it was impossible to ignore the twenty pounds of weight that she had gained since returning home. Joanne kept up with her five-mile runs, but she was now concerned enough to consult her family doctor. "I thought it was just weight gain, but I went to see my local doctor who took one look at me and said, 'Joanne, you have ascites.' I didn't know what that was at the time. He did an ultrasound, which I was told showed a cyst, so he referred me to my gynecologist."

The term "ascites" dates back as far as the fourth century BC, when Hippocrates described the condition. He used the Greek word *askos*, meaning a leather bag or sheepskin used to carry wine, water, or oil. Hippocrates realized that not only was ascites directly related to a diseased liver but it was also likely to be fatal. In one of his famous aphorisms, Hippocrates wrote, "When the liver is filled with water and bursts into [the omentum], in this case the belly is filled with water and the patient dies." A century later, Erasistratos of Chios proposed a mechanistic explanation, writing that ascites was "a chronic and scirrhous inflammation of the liver or spleen, which prevents the assimilation of the food in the bowels and its distribution through the body, but changes it into water, which being refrigerated, is deposited between the intestine and the peritoneum." Some aspects of this description remain essentially accurate today.

In modern language, ascites is the abnormal accumulation of fluid inside the abdominal, or peritoneal, cavity. It has numerous causes, but the symptoms are fairly uniform: a distended abdomen, weight gain, and sometimes swelling in the legs. When the ascites is large enough, it presses on the diaphragm and patients feel short of breath. The peritoneal cavity is normally a potential space that exists between the lining of the abdominal wall (called the peritoneum) and the organs that occupy the abdomen. These organs lie right up against the abdominal wall, and other than a tiny amount of fluid that can be normal, there is no "space." When fluid begins to accumulate, which it can do for many different reasons, it is called ascites. One of the most important as well as most common causes is liver disease. The liver, a large solid organ located in the right upper quadrant of the abdomen, is a complex chemical factory. The raw materials are the by-products delivered to the liver from the last meal from the intestines. The finished products are the usable building blocks to be metabolized or stored elsewhere in the body.

Because of this critical function, the liver has two independent sources of blood flow. The first is the hepatic artery. This vessel brings oxygen-rich blood from the heart to the liver. The second source of blood is from the portal vein. Everywhere else in the body, the veins carry blood away from a tissue and back to the heart, but the portal vein is unique. It does drain blood away from a tissue—the intestines—but the blood does not flow straight back to the heart. The portal vein first delivers all the nutrients from the intestines to the liver. The liver processes these chemical substrates, storing some of the result in the form of glycogen and packaging the rest to be distributed to other parts of the body, such as fat and muscle. These chemical building blocks that the liver manufactures (triglycerides, free fatty acids, and amino acids) are then drained away from the liver and back to the heart by the hepatic vein. Thus, two vessels bring blood to the liver—the hepatic artery and the portal vein—and one vessel, the hepatic vein, drains blood from the liver back to the heart.

In certain forms of liver disease, the blood that flows into the liver is partially blocked from leaving. This can occur from liver scarring in cirrhosis (the "scirrhous inflammation" of Erasistratos) or liver fibrosis, or from a blockage of the hepatic vein. When the venous pressure in the liver builds up, the lymph from the surface of the liver begins to "sweat" into the abdominal cavity. Heart failure is another cause of this same kind of ascites. If the heart is not pumping effectively, the blood backs up in the hepatic vein and the same train of events is triggered. Another cause of blood backing up is when the hepatic vein clots or becomes otherwise obstructed. In each of these situations, the result of backed-up plumbing is called portal hypertension, or increased pressure in the portal vein. One manifestation of portal hypertension is ascites.

Another cause of ascites is infection in the peritoneal cavity. In past centuries, tuberculosis was an important cause of infectious ascites. Today, peritonitis caused by normal bacteria that live in the intestine and cross over into the abdomen is the most common infection. Sometimes this occurs spontaneously in the presence of liver disease, other times after the perforation from appendicitis or some other abdominal catastrophe.

Cancer, particularly mesothelioma related to asbestos exposure, and metastatic cells from ovarian cancer, are relatively common causes of ascites. Just about any cancer can spread to the peritoneum and lead to ascites.

To diagnose the specific cause of ascites, doctors perform a simple procedure that has been used since the time of Hippocrates. The procedure is called paracentesis. After cleaning the skin with an antibacterial solution and anesthetizing it (two upgrades since the fourth century BC), the physician inserts a sterile needle directly into the abdomen. Fluid is withdrawn into a syringe, after which it is analyzed in the laboratory to test the protein level and to look for microorganisms or cancer cells.

Joanne was hospitalized in May for a battery of tests to determine the cause of her ascites. There were the usual perfunctory blood and urine tests; some showed trivial abnormalities like a slightly low protein level and a slightly high enzyme (called the LDH) level, but nothing of any diagnostic consequence. She was subjected to a nuclear isotope liver-spleen scan, an ultrasound exam, and even a liver biopsy. This test showed some mild fibrosis, but again, nothing diagnostic. She then had an upper GI series and finally a paracentesis to directly test the ascites fluid. The ultrasound showed a probable fibroid tumor in her uterus, but this was thought to be a benign growth that was unrelated to her symptoms. Despite the thoroughness of the testing during her ten-day hospitalization, there were no definitive results.

She did not like being cooped up in a hospital; she could neither eat nor exercise the way she was used to. Young remembers, "I was like a mad woman. I missed the exercise. All I wanted to do was get out of the hospital. I was practically running up and down the hallways. And my doctor wasn't into nutrition. He was surprised at all the vitamins I was taking. In fact, I had to smuggle them into the hospital. I felt like I was doing drugs."

After all the tests came back negative, she was discharged. Several days later, she went to her gynecologist, who was still concerned about the possibility of ovarian cancer, so he wanted to schedule a more invasive test—a laparoscopy. This procedure, now commonplace, was relatively new back in 1981. A surgeon inserts a rigid metal tube through a small incision in the abdomen, and through the tube it is possible to examine the contents of the abdomen and perform some surgical procedures.

Joanne recalls that visit vividly. "I wasn't thrilled, obviously. My daughter was with me; she was pregnant at the time. We left the doctor's office and went out to lunch to discuss all the 'what if's.' I decided that if I had cancer, I was going to fight it with everything I had."

The laparoscopy was done on June 8, 1981. The procedure itself went smoothly. "He told me everything looked fine," recalls Young. Three days later, however, she received a phone call from the doctor. The news wasn't good. "He was my daughter's obstetrician at the time and one of my running partners. His voice was all broken up. He said, 'I don't know how to tell you this, Joanne, but we found some cancer cells.' He referred me to a gynecologic cancer specialist in Boston, Dr. Thomas Leavitt, who practiced at the Brigham and Woman's Hospital." After examining her, Leavitt ordered another round of tests. She underwent a barium enema, an abdominal CT scan, a D&C (a gynecologic procedure to test for uterine cancer), mammograms, and endoscopic examinations of the lower intestine and bladder.

All of the tests were negative; there was no evidence of a malignancy. However, the doctors in Boston decided to do another paracentesis, and yet again, Joanne's ascites fluid revealed cancer cells.

It was now August. To try to get to the bottom of the problem in the most definitive manner, Dr. Leavitt scheduled open abdominal surgery to directly inspect the internal organs. This approach would allow him to biopsy and remove any suspicious tissue. The surgery went without a hitch. The findings: no cancer, and somewhat surprisingly, no cancer cells in the abdominal fluid.

Yet the fluid, which had receded somewhat over a three-month period, was beginning to accumulate again. "And I was starting to feel lousy and weak," Joanne recalls. "After a while, I couldn't run or even bike; the pressure from the fluid made it hard to breathe. At one hospital visit, they drained four and a half quarts of fluid through a catheter. Six weeks after the abdominal surgery, I felt terrible."

In September, Young was referred to yet another physician, Dr. Charles Trey, who was a gastroenterologist and a liver specialist at the nearby New England Deaconess Hospital. Joanne had so much fluid that it was beginning to accumulate around her lungs, and she was no longer the picture of health. Dr. Trey remembers her as a "bubbly and vivacious woman," but her physical health had flagged severely and an excerpt from his clinical notes reads, "She was cachectic [emaciated] with a markedly distended abdomen. . . . There was obvious wasting of her temporal muscles and her eyes were sunken."

"She was very health conscious," recalls Trey, "but I was concerned because she used so many vitamins and enzymes and herbal teas. I first thought the problem might be vitamin A toxicity." Excess vitamin A sometimes causes a liver problem, but blood tests eliminated that possibility. Looking for all sorts of unusual diagnoses, Trey tested for excess copper, iron, mercury, and zinc, and for diseases with names like paroxysmal nocturnal hemoglobinuria and porphyria. All were normal. To help improve her breathing, he removed more fluid from the abdomen, and this time he also removed fluid from around her right lung. He tested the fluid for tuberculosis and other infections—again, with negative results.

Trey did, however, solve one mystery: the reason for the cancer diagnosis. The cells that twice had been interpreted as malignant were the large cells that line the abdominal cavity, called mesothelial cells. When these mesothelial cells become inflamed, they can change their shape and appearance under the microscope and mimic cancer cells. On careful reexamination, they proved to be completely benign.

Although the possibility of cancer had been eliminated, there was still no diagnosis. Dr. Trey now thought that the leading possibility was a condition called the Budd-Chiari syndrome.

Budd-Chiari syndrome applies to a group of disorders, the common denominator of which is obstruction of outflow from the liver (blockage of the hepatic vein) that results in severe ascites. The first report of this condition, in 1845, is ascribed to Dr. George Budd, a distinguished physician who practiced in London. He wrote extensively on disorders of the liver, although his contribution to this entity was relatively minor. In 1899, the Austrian pathologist Hans Chiari published the first pathological description of the entity that now bears his name.

Most cases are caused by a blood clot in the major hepatic vein, but there are many other causes. In fact, in Chiari's original report, he wrote about an inflammatory process that resulted in clotting of the small veins draining the liver, not the large hepatic vein itself. The increased pressure in the liver leads to portal hypertension, which in turn results in ascites.

Trying to establish a diagnosis of Budd-Chiari syndrome, Dr. Trey repeated a liver biopsy, this time getting a deeper sample of tissue. The findings were supportive of a diagnosis of Budd-Chiari, but not conclusive. Nowadays, a simple CT scan could make the diagnosis, but this was 1981, so Dr. Trey ordered a hepatic venogram, a specialized x-ray procedure in which a catheter is threaded into one of the larger veins in the body—the vena cava—and then dye is injected into the hepatic vein. The dye outlines the veins themselves, and the doctor can also measure pressures in the veins. Any large clot in the hepatic vein will be visible. The pressure measurements confirmed Trey's suspicions, but there was no large clot. So while he had unraveled one more layer of the enigma—his patient had Budd-Chiari syndrome—he still lacked a specific diagnosis. What was causing the high portal pressures in Joanne Young's liver?

Budd-Chiari syndrome is usually caused by disorders that are characterized by a tendency for blood to clot too easily, and Dr. Trey's workup tested for all of these conditions, but those tests also proved negative. At this point, the list of potential causes of the problem was growing thin.

Young's condition was also deteriorating, and the need for treatment was becoming increasingly urgent. Trey next consulted with Dr. William V. McDermott, a professor of surgery at the Harvard Medical School and chief of surgery at the Deaconess Hospital. Both physicians agreed that to prevent liver failure, Joanne needed surgery to halt the inexorable progression of the ascites. The kind of surgery they proposed, called a porto-caval shunt, is basically a sophisticated plumbing job that shunts the blood away from the high pressure portal system into the low pressure vena cava.

Shortly afterward, McDermott performed the surgery to reduce the pressure in her portal vein. The surgery was successful. Recalls McDermott, "That cleared up her ascites as you would it expect it would, but post-operatively, I was really baffled as to what could have caused this." The patient was discharged, feeling markedly improved but still without a complete understanding of what was causing her problem. Not too long after the surgery, in December 1981, nine months after her symptoms first began, Young suffered from a brief complication called hepatic encephalopathy, a state of confusion that results when the body tries to process large amounts of protein that is bypassing the liver by way of the shunt that McDermott had created.

With treatment, the encephalopathy rapidly cleared up, but early in 1982, McDermott and Trey remained mystified by the cause of the inflammation of Joanne's liver. One day, the two doctors and a Harvard medical student who was involved in Young's care, Paul Ridker, were reviewing the case and discussing the various herbal preparations that Joanne had been taking. That is when they got the final clue needed to solve the mystery. Trey had observed from the very beginning that Young was an avid consumer of herbal and natural products. He and

McDermott remembered an obscure study published almost thirty years earlier, about Jamaicans with an atypical pattern of liver disease—and a diet that included herbal tea.

In the 1950s, a doctor noticed an unusual liver problem in Jamaicans who drank "bush teas"—concoctions prepared using various wild plants. Physicians from the University College of Medicine in Jamaica reported a series of five cases of an odd form of liver disease with prominent ascites. The patients were children (the oldest was eighteen), and their liver biopsies showed findings strikingly similar to that described in Chiari's original work. These children had all been drinking bush teas, which contained various plants. These investigators suggested that substances in the bush tea were causing the liver disease.

A far larger epidemic of approximately sixteen hundred cases occurred in Afghanistan in the early 1970s. The report from the *Lancet*, published in 1976, goes as follows:

> *During 1970–1972, the north-western region of Afghanistan was hit by severe drought. The brunt of the calamity fell on the district of Gulran, affecting a population of about 35,000 in 98 villages. The district consists of undulating hills with scanty vegetation serving as pasturelands. Water is scarce and obtained from shallow wells and small springs. Communications are very poor, and during the winter the villages are snowbound and totally isolated. The inhabitants are illiterate and the principal occupation is farming. Their diet consists of wheat bread and occasional meat. During the years of drought, the flocks of sheep and goats were mostly destroyed, and there was a serious shortage of food.*
>
> *Toward the middle of 1974, cases of huge abdominal distention and emaciation started to appear in the villages and soon assumed epidemic proportions. The poorest families were disproportionately involved. In many instances, several members in a family were affected within weeks of each other and all had died.*

The illness began gradually, with loss of appetite, fatigue, and muscle wasting. Most of the patients had enlarged livers and massive ascites. Nearly 25 percent of the region's population developed liver disease, and many died, since access to medical care in the area was poor. In villagers who were investigated at a hospital, the liver specimens showed the same findings as in the Jamaican children who drank the bush tea, and in autopsy material from some of the fatal cases, the doctors found the same occlusive disease of the small veins that Chiari had described.

As for the cause of the epidemic, an important clue emerged from one of the villagers. This man, a shepherd, had observed the same effects on his flock of sheep, which he had fed some of his wheat crop that was overgrown by a weed. When he went to slaughter the sheep, he found that most of the animals had shrunken, scarred livers and large amounts of ascites. From the beginning, the researchers thought the disease was most likely caused by some sort of toxic exposure. They fairly quickly ruled out chemical fertilizers, preservatives, and pesticides. Because of the shepherd's testimony and because of the appearance of the liver lesions, the possibility of contaminated plants immediately became a serious one.

A plant called *Heliotropium* was found to be growing in the wheat fields, and when the grain was harvested, the *Heliotropium* had been gathered along with it. The wheat was then ground into flour, the *Heliotropium* seeds were pulverized too, and the bread made from the wheat unintentionally included *Heliotropium* flour. Families that had cleaned out the intruding plants from the wheat did not develop liver disease. In the other families, there were often several members who were affected simultaneously.

The researchers examined the wheat and calculated that about three hundred milligrams of *Heliotropium* seeds had made their way into every kilogram of wheat. Analysis of the *Heliotropium* plant showed substances called pyrrolizidine alkaloids, which cause inflammation of the small hepatic veins, one cause of the Budd-Chiari syndrome. Hundreds of plant species contain these toxic alkaloids, but most come from those known as *Senecio*, *Crotalaria*, and *Heliotropium*.

The first reported case of veno-occlusive disease of the liver, in South Africa in 1920, was caused by eating bread contaminated with *Senecio* plants; veterinarians have diagnosed the same problem in livestock since the 1950s. In the mid-1970s in India, a moderately large outbreak of Budd-Chiari syndrome was nearly a carbon copy of the Afghan epidemic. This one occurred in the drought-prone Sarguja district in north-central India, where 486 people lived in four villages. The dietary staple is a cereal called *gondli*. The cereal in the district became contaminated with a wild plant of the *Crotalaria* group, and an investigation was begun after some villagers developed ascites and swollen livers. Of the sixty-seven affected villagers, twenty-eight died (a mortality rate of 42 percent). The specimens from liver biopsies as well as examination by autopsy of the fatal cases were all consistent with veno-occlusive disease of the liver.

More recently, in Iraq in 1993, a family of Bedouins living near the city of Mosul placed some of their grain under their dwellings, a traditional practice for storing grain to be consumed later, during the winter. As in the Afghanistan epidemic, the Bedouins had unwittingly mixed some *Senecio* weeds in with the wheat. During the winter of 1994, fourteen of them were admitted to the hospital with massive ascites and enlarged livers; two of them died.

Budd-Chiari syndrome from veno-occlusive disease brought on by these toxic alkaloids is not only a third-world phenomenon, and it is not only related to inadvertent consumption of tainted grains. In 1976, a twenty-six-year-old transplant to Britain from the Caribbean islands developed ascites and liver disease. She was found to be "addicted" to maté, a Paraguayan tea that she had been taking for years made from the leaves of various species of *Ilex* plants. After two liver biopsies and finally a portal shunt procedure, she ultimately died from her disease. Samples of this maté tea, both bought at stores as well as some that was owned by the woman, tested positive for pyrrolizidine alkaloids.

Not long thereafter, reports were published of two Arizona infants who died from liver disease after they were given herbal teas for a cough. The first case was that of a six-month-old Latino girl who was admitted to a Tucson hospital because of vomiting and irritability. Two weeks earlier the child had visited the pediatrician for a probable upper respiratory viral infection. On admission to the hospital, the child had an enlarged liver and massive ascites. A liver biopsy and other test results were consistent with veno-occlusive disease of the liver. On questioning, the child's parents admitted to feeding her large quantities of a tea prepared from a local herb called gordolobo yerba. When the tea was analyzed in the laboratory, it was found that the tea was in fact made from a *Senecio* plant.

The second case was that of a two-month-old infant admitted to a Phoenix hospital for a one-day history of lethargy and vomiting. The doctors found massive ascites and liver damage. Despite intensive therapy, the child died. The parents had been giving the child an herbal preparation for a cough. The tea was sold at a local pharmacy; on analysis, it was found to contain the same *Senecio* plant as in the other Arizona case.

The common denominator among these deadly plants and herbs was that they all contained a toxin from the group called pyrrolizidine alkaloids. These substances cause inflammation of the hepatic veins that drain blood away from the liver and back to the heart. They can lead to potentially deadly scarring and obstruction of venous flow. Despite these cases, the concept of a Budd-Chiari syndrome from a toxic plant was still off the radar screen of most physicians in 1982. In a lengthy review of the syndrome published in a major journal in that year, only a few sentences were devoted to the subject of the plants.

Aware of the Jamaican bush tea episode and now focused on their patient's penchant for herbal teas and natural remedies, the Harvard doctors and their student were intrigued that this might be the potential link to her condition. As a medical student, Ridker had the most time on his hands. Young recalls that he "asked me to bring everything that I used."

After the patient complied, Ridker reviewed exactly what herbal preparations Joanne was taking. "There was a long list," he recalls. "I went around to the various health food stores where she shopped and bought the different preparations that she used. Then I spent days at Harvard Medical School's botany library trying to identify the substances."

There were, as it turned out, two suspicious preparations: a tea called MU-16 and comfrey-pepsin capsules. Because she enjoyed the taste so much, Joanne had been drinking three cups of tea per day for about six months before first seeing her doctor in April 1981. She had also been taking two of the capsules with each meal, to help digestion. The doctors sent samples of these preparations to Dr. Ryan Huxtable, a pharmacologist in Arizona with special expertise in pyrrolizidine alkaloid toxicity. The MU-16 tea, which was supposed to be ginseng, contained large amounts of pyrrolizidine alkaloids. Samples from different lots purchased at different times contained varying amounts of the toxic alkaloids, suggesting poor quality control by the manufacturer. The comfrey-pepsin capsules contained even larger amounts of the toxic alkaloids.

Unwittingly, Joanne Young had been poisoning herself over the four months before she got ill. She had been drinking as much as a quart of the MU-16 per day, in addition to taking six capsules of the comfrey-pepsin.

She is not the only patient to suffer serious side effects from comfrey. In 1986, a thirteen-year-old boy with inflammatory bowel disease decided to go off the medications prescribed by his physicians and started using acupuncture and ingesting large quantities of tea prepared from comfrey root. In June of that year, he developed profound fatigue, weight loss, and abdominal pain. His liver swelled and he developed massive ascites.

In 1978, a New York social worker consulted a homeopathic doctor because of allergies and feelings of fatigue. The doctor recommended comfrey tea. Four years later, blood tests showed mild abnormalities in her liver. Four years after that, in 1986, she developed ascites. Paracentesis was nondiagnostic, and the ascites persisted. Like Joanne Young, the social worker also required a surgical shunt to treat her intractable ascites. Her liver specialist saw her drinking herbal tea while she was being admitted for the shunt treatment. When he witnessed this, according to the patient, "It was like a light bulb went off in his head. He almost yelled at me, 'Don't take that stuff; it could ruin your liver.' I was taking quite a bit of it." Like Young, once the diagnosis was established, she stopped taking the comfrey and recovered.

Comfrey, *Symphytum officinale*, is a perennial bush native to Europe and Asia. The plant grows to between two and five feet tall, with oblong leaves and dull purple or white flowers that bloom in tight clusters. The root is fleshy and filled with a white liquid. Its roots and leaves contain a substance called allantoin, which has been used to maintain healthy skin and to treat pulled muscles and ligaments as well as sprains and fractures. People use it both as a topical ointment and as an oral preparation.

There is no scientific data to support any of these uses. At the time that Joanne Young was taking her comfrey, the herb was completely unregulated. Because comfrey was on the market prior to 1958, when legislation governing food additives was passed, it was exempt from FDA regulations.

It is also difficult to know exactly what one is consuming in comfrey and other herbal preparations. For one thing, many of these potions are not standardized like typical pharmaceuticals. Batches of teas made from leaves of plants can be contaminated with other plants, and leaves harvested in one season may differ considerably in their active ingredients from those harvested at another time of year.

There is also the risk of simple misidentification. One elderly couple from Washington state went to a health spa, where it was recommended that they drink comfrey tea for their arthritis. So they went hunting for natural comfrey in the forest. On May 7, 1977, the wife picked some plants that she believed were comfrey and brewed a tea, which they both drank. Within an hour, they were both seized by nausea, vomiting, dizziness, and sweating.

The husband, who knew more about plants than his wife, went to the refrigerator a few hours later and realized that the leaves were not comfrey at all, but foxglove. This plant, which superficially resembles comfrey, is the source of the powerful cardiac drug digitalis. He immediately called an ambulance, but by the time it arrived, his wife was dead. The husband made it to the hospital, but despite intensive treatment, he too died less than a day later.

Herbal remedies are a $1.8 billion industry in the United States alone. There is a general notion that if a substance is natural, or herbal, then it must be safe; this is clearly a misconception. Many different herbal preparations have serious health risks. Some lead to problems with blood coagulation. Others lead to acute hepatitis and gastroenteritis. Still others cause lethal cardiac conditions, and others lead to neurological symptoms. Many of them can be fatal. There are numerous case reports of herbs that have led to serious health consequences. One involved a life-threatening allergic reaction to chamomile. Another was the case of a newborn that died from veno-occlusive disease of the liver related to herbal tea her mother consumed during pregnancy.

Not long after the incident with Joanne, Dr. Ridker, now a professor at Harvard himself, said, "Nobody should drink comfrey. Even small amounts can have disastrous effects. There is just no risk to benefit ratio." In July 2001, more than a decade after Joanne Young nearly died from using it, the FDA banned all oral comfrey preparations. Its advisory reads: "[The] FDA believes that the available scientific information is sufficient to firmly establish that dietary supplements that contain comfrey or any other source of pyrrolizidine alkaloids are adulterated. . . . The agency strongly recommends that firms marketing a product containing comfrey or another source of pyrrolizidine alkaloids remove the product from the market and alert its customers to immediately stop using the product. The agency advises that it is prepared to use its authority and resources to remove products from the market." Many other countries have taken the same step.

As soon as the doctors learned the cause of Joanne's liver ailment, they strongly recommended that she stop consuming comfrey, the substance that she had been taking to improve her health. She complied, of course, and she is now in good health—and shows no trace whatsoever of ascites. As for her penchant for herbal teas, she will enjoy a cup of chamomile tea from time to time. During the summer, she may have a glass of Red Zinger. Otherwise, she's off herbs.

It all started as a perfectly routine case. Luisa Alvarez-Ruiz (as I'll call her) was a five-year-old girl whose family brought her to the emergency department because of a headache. Among the long list of symptoms that bring patients to a doctor's attention, headache is one of the most common. So the doctors began asking their usual questions and taking their normal measurements. However, they did not find anything particularly worrisome in the responses and metrics, and her physical examination seemed to be normal. But for some reason, in part because Luisa's headaches had been present for a few months, the first pediatric emergency physicians who were taking care of Luisa were anxious; that sixth sense that all good doctors have was registering concern.

Head pain is nearly ubiquitous in human beings, and it is a rare individual who has never experienced a headache at some point. The vast majority of headaches are not severe in the sense that, if untreated, they will not cause death or loss of neurological or visual function. Most of these patients have tension-related or migraine headaches. These two "primary" headache disorders are incredibly common; the annual incidence of migraine alone in the general population is approximately 12 percent, and even higher in women. The lifetime incidence of migraine ranges from about 18 percent in men to 45 percent in women. Of course most of these patients never end up in an emergency room for these headaches.

But some do. One would expect that patients whose headaches are severe enough to bring them to an emergency department would have more serious causes, but even in this group, only about 5 percent of them are diagnosed with a life- or brain-threatening problem. When a patient with a headache does come to the hospital, the physician first goes through a series of questions designed to establish a particular diagnosis. Did the pain start abruptly or gradually? How severe is the pain? Is it the worst that the patient has ever had? Is the quality of the pain similar to prior episodes? Is there associated fever, or vomiting or any new neurological symptoms? After factoring in the answers to these and other questions, the physician will then perform a physical examination, again hoping to pinpoint the cause. The vast majority of migraine and tension headache sufferers have normal physical exams. By the end of the history and the physical, patients usually fall into one of three groups.

At one extreme is the group that has no worrisome features. The headache sounds familiar to prior episodes or the characteristics are classic for migraine or tension syndromes; the physical examination is normal. These patients need treatment for their pain and follow-up with their primary care doctor. On the other extreme is a group with obvious, clear-cut worrisome findings. They have a new onset of a worst-ever unusual headache, or perhaps a new abnormality in their neurological examination, a high fever, or some other symptom or sign that strongly suggests a serious problem. The decision-making in this group is easy; these patients need further testing and treatment until the source of the finding is explained. And then there are patients who fall into a third, intermediate group. When the doctor factors in all the information available, the patients simply do not fall neatly into the first or the second group. The need to do further testing is ambiguous.

Most of the patients in this last group turn out to have simple problems that do not threaten their vision, brain, or life. A few, however, will have serious neurological dangers that need to be addressed, and which, if not diagnosed and treated properly, can end catastrophically.

Sometimes, in ambiguous cases, a doctor will decide to do further testing, just to be safe. Other times, he or she may simply arrange a follow-up appointment with the person's primary care physician in the next few days and use time as a diagnostic tool. One other "test" that is sometimes available is a consultation with a specialist, such as a neurologist. This is what the emergency physicians decided to do in Luisa's case.

"That was the point where I became involved," recalls Dr. David Urion, a pediatric neurologist at Boston's prestigious Children's Hospital. "She came to the ED [emergency department] complaining of this headache that lasted for several months. The ED staff had already evaluated her but did not come up with a diagnosis. What they found was that the pain itself was fairly nondescript. The headache was 'all over' but more in the front and behind the eyes. It seemed to be a 'pressure' and it began very insidiously a few months ago. She was Latina and was accompanied by a hoard of family members—both of the parents, her grandmother, and a few cousins. The relatives did not seem to know exactly what we meant when we used the word 'headache.'

"The pain was constant over time but seemed to wax and wane over the course of the day. She had some sensitivity to light, but there were no clear things that made the headache better or worse. She also had some nausea but no vomiting. They also had determined that there was no history of head trauma and no recent illnesses that seemed relevant. Also there was no family history of headaches in general, and specifically, no family history of migraine.

"Developmentally she was normal. One other thing that the family noticed was that she seemed clumsy and that she was bumping into things lately. When the doctors in the ED did their physical examination, it was normal. Specifically her neurological examination was normal. The ED staff was properly concerned so they asked for a neurology consult," recalls Dr. Urion, sitting in his neatly kept office on a top floor of a stately marble and granite building on the quadrangle of Harvard Medical School. Although Luisa's case had occurred several years before the interview, it stood out in Urion's memory such that he remembered the minute details with remarkable clarity.

Urion continues, "One question that all the doctors asked was, 'did she take any medications?' She did not. The only other piece of history that the neurology fellow obtained that the ED staff had not was an unusual social circumstance. The child lived with the parents in Boston every other month, and on the alternate months, she lived with her grandmother in New York, the Bronx I think.

"The ED fellow got a negative exam and the ED attending got a negative exam. The neurology resident also got a normal exam, and I found no venous pulsations (all had looked), but no frank papilledema."

Papilledema is an ominous finding indeed. Checking the eyes is an important part of the neurological examination, especially in headache patients. Doctors look at the lids to see if they droop, and check the pupils to see if their reaction to bright light is normal. They ask the patients to look to the right and then to the left, up and down, to check the nerves that control the muscles that move the eyes. And they look at the retina using an ophthalmoscope. This instrument was invented in 1851 and both literally and figuratively opened up an entire new diagnostic world for physicians. The ophthalmoscope is the small cylindrical hand-held instrument that the doctor holds close to the patient's eye—within a half an inch or so—and then shines a light into the retina. The scope is designed so that the path of light and the aperture through which the physician looks are perfectly aligned, allowing a view of the retina.

This ability is exceedingly important. In terms of vision, the retina is where the rubber meets the road. When photons of light strike the nerve cells of the retina, the physical energy of the light is transformed into electrical energy in the retina's rod and cone cells, and the electrical impulses are transmitted via the optic nerve to an area in the back of the brain called the occipital lobes. Here, the signals are interpreted, and that is how we see objects.

In the developing embryo, the retina grows from the brain, so it is ac-tually nerve tissue, a part of the central nervous system. When doctors look at the retina, they are examining a part of the brain itself. The poets say that looking in the eyes offers a window to the soul; for doctors, quite literally the retina is a window to the brain. The veins and arteries of the retina will often show the same changes as the veins and arteries of the brain itself. The central portion of the retina is called the optic disc. This is the place where the nerve fibers of the optic nerve enter the eye; because the bundles of fibers are large, there is a slight raised area, which is called the papilla.

Papilledema is swelling (edema) of this area of the central retina and is a sign of elevated intracranial pressure.

Because the brain lies in a tight bony box—the skull—directly mea-suring the pressure of the brain within the cranium (intracranial pres-sure) involves surgically placing a metal pressure gauge through a hole drilled into the skull. Looking at the papilla of the retina, however, will sometimes allow doctors to diagnose high intracranial pressure without such a drastic step. Some patients, though, have elevated pressure in the head without having papilledema. In those cases, the veins of the retina will supply a clue, albeit a very subtle one. The veins of the retina will normally pulsate with the heartbeat. The loss of these normal pulsations can be a clue that there may be raised intracranial pressure.

Although Luisa did not have papilledema, Dr. Urion, the most experienced of the physicians who examined her, could not see any venous pulsations. Without frank papilledema, there was no way to know if the absence of venous pulsations indicated a problem or not, but it was just one more piece of a puzzle that suggested the possibility that Luisa's headache was not a minor, primary headache disorder.

"She had already been scheduled for a head CT scan by about this time," Urion remembers, "and the scan was done and was interpreted as normal. But there still seemed to be something amiss." This is an example of an experienced clinician following a gut instinct, a factor that cannot be measured or quantified, but something that every doctor understands. For this reason, the team persisted in the evaluation. Fortunately, the patient had come in during the morning of a weekday, which made some options more easily available than during off hours. So after some discussion with the neuroradiologists, the clinicians finally persuaded them to perform a second brain scan: a magnetic resonance imaging study.

As good as a CT scan is, the MRI, especially of the brain, is a far superior imaging technique. It takes longer and is less readily available in many parts of the country and times of the day, but it shows detailed anatomy of the brain that the CT does not. The MRI is also much better in looking at the backmost reaches of the brain—the posterior fossa—which is where the cerebellum lies. The cerebellum is the part of the brain responsible for coordinated movement and balance.

"The main thing I was concerned about was the possibility of missing some process in the posterior fossa, perhaps an infiltrating tumor," said Urion, "because recall that she had the history of bumping into things and clumsiness. Finally the radiologists agreed to do the MRI and they used gadolinium, a contrast agent that might better define a tumor if that was the problem.

"The initial report showed 'something funny.' There was a group of neuroradiologists huddled around the scans as if in Talmudic discussion.

The films were in front of them and they were discussing the results," recalled Dr. Urion.

Patients, victims of television shows about doctors, often think that x-rays and CT scans and MRI scans show clear-cut black-and-white results. A given diagnosis either is established or is excluded. Unfortunately for all involved, this simply is not the case. Some interpretation is necessary. Even after performing one of the most sophisticated brain imaging studies known, and even though some of the brightest and most experienced pediatric radiologists in the world were looking at the images, there remained a significant amount of ambiguity after these studies were done.

To have an MRI, the patient is placed on a stretcher that moves inside a large cylindrical and very powerful magnet. Before sending a patient into an MRI machine, technicians go through a meticulous checklist to make sure that there is no metal in the patient's body—a heart pacemaker or a small piece of metal from prior trauma. All the medical equipment in the room is free of ferrous metals. Otherwise, when the magnet is turned on, any of these objects could move inside the patient's body or fly through the room. Serious accidents and injuries have occurred from both of those situations.

The scientific basis for the MRI is that water molecules are affected by magnetic energy. Small differences in water content in adjacent tissues, or between normal tissue and abnormal tissue, will appear different on an MRI. To the trained eye, these subtle differences are the hallmark of diagnosis. Slight shades of gray can have enormous diagnostic significance, but slight shades of gray are also open to interpretation. One person's gray is another's white or black. Increasingly, radiologists are no longer working with hard copies of x-ray (or CT or MRI) films anymore; the images are digitized and then viewed on high-tech computer work stations.

When Urion went back to the radiology department after the MRI had been done, he saw that "they were moving the cursor back and forth and playing with the knobs and the dials on the screen to measure the pixels and adjust the contrast. The 'something funny' turned out to be some enhancement [showing a brighter signal] of both optic nerves. So we asked for an ophthalmology consultation, and they agreed and said send her up to the clinic, where we have all of the equipment and it will be easier to test her. Well, when the ophthalmologist fellow called back on the phone with his report, you could almost hear him grinning like the Cheshire cat over the phone. He said to us, 'Did you know your patient is almost blind, doctor?'"

Luisa's visual acuity was 20/400 in the left eye, and there was almost no vision in the right eye. "Well, now we had an explanation for her bumping into things. But beyond the extremely poor vision, they didn't find anything precise on the retina exam. They just thought that it looked 'funny,' but they could not diagnose any particular ophthalmologic problem."

By mid-afternoon, Luisa had already undergone an extensive evaluation—a neurology consultation, an ophthalmology consultation, a CT scan, and an MRI scan. The only thing she still lacked was the most important of all—a diagnosis. Dr. Urion decided to examine the brain in the one way that they had not so far. They would do a lumbar puncture, or spinal tap.

The first lumbar puncture was performed in 1891 by a German neurologist, Heinrich Quincke. Even in that era there was a robust dissemination of medical information, and Dr. Arthur Wentworth soon performed the procedure in the United States, at Boston Children's Hospital, on a two-year-old girl who was thought to have tuberculosis of the brain. He described the procedure: "We punctured the spinal canal . . . and withdrew six cubic centimeters of a clear fluid which looked like distilled water. No TB bacilli were found. . . . Immediately after tapping the canal, the child became restless, throwing herself about the bed, clutching at her hair, and giving vent to short cries. The pulse rose to over 250 per minute, the respiration was superficial, and the skin was cool and slightly livid. Subcutaneous injections of brandy and ether were given, heaters applied, and the foot of the bed raised. The condition persisted about the same for three-quarters of an hour, and then the child became quieter."

As tests go, it is not a favorite of patients. But it is a very safe and usually easily accomplished procedure, Dr. Wentworth's harrowing experience notwithstanding. After cleaning and anesthetizing the lumbar area, a doctor places a needle into the patient's back. The needle is angled in such a way as to go between adjacent bones of the spine and enter the subarachnoid space, where cerebrospinal fluid resides. Among a number of other functions, this fluid acts as a shock absorber in head trauma and serves some nutritive role for the brain and spinal cord. It is important for patients to know that the needle is inserted several inches below where the spinal cord itself ends, and serious side effects from a lumbar puncture are extraordinarily rare.

When the doctor performs this procedure, a specimen of the spinal fluid, which is normally crystal clear like water, is sent to the lab to be tested for cells, chemical composition (such as protein and glucose levels), and the presence of microorganisms, among other things. The doctor usually also measures the pressure of the spinal fluid, as this is one way to directly gauge the intracranial pressure. The fluid from Luisa was clear like water. The protein and glucose were normal. There were no abnormal cells or bacteria. But the pressure was two and a half times the normal level.

"So now we had a diagnosis, but it was a diagnosis that only raised another series of questions," recalls Dr. Urion. "She had pseudotumor cerebri. To have that diagnosis in a skinny five-year-old was pretty unusual in itself."

Pseudotumor cerebri comes from Latin, meaning "false tumor of the brain." A few years after the first lumbar puncture, Heinrich Quincke and another eminent German neurologist, Max Nonne, discovered this entity, although earlier case reports of patients that seem to have had the problem predated their seminal work. One of Nonne's distinctions is that he was among the four physicians who attended Vladimir Lenin, architect of Russia's Bolshevik revolution, who had a series of strokes that led to his death in 1924. Quincke and Nonne knew that most patients with the combination of papilledema (seen through the ophthalmoscope) and elevated intracranial pressure (measured with the lumbar puncture) had a mass—tumor, abscess, or blood clot—causing these findings. Both men documented patients who had papilledema and elevated intracranial pressure without an obvious cause (no tumor, abscess, or other cause was found). These patients did not die, and in fact many improved over time.

These doctors were working long before CT scans and MRI tests, so there was no way for them to find these masses until autopsy. But Quincke and Nonne noticed that sometimes the improvement in these patients (often younger ones who seemed to have a tumor, but did not) seemed to follow one or more lumbar punctures. Because the patients didn't actually have tumors, Nonne applied the name pseudotumor cerebri. Although it is clear that some of the cases these men described did not have what we would today call pseudotumor cerebri, many of them did.

The exact mechanism for this condition was unknown to Quincke and Nonne, but they hypothesized that it had to do with the flow of cerebrospinal fluid. Over a century later, doctors still do not precisely know the cause of the problem. More modern names for the condition are idiopathic intracranial hypertension—doctor-speak for increased pressure in the head for reasons that nobody understands—and benign intracranial hypertension, which points to the overall good outcomes. Whatever the cause, and despite these more modern descriptions, Nonne's nomenclature stuck and remains in common use today.

The large majority of patients with pseudotumor cerebri have the finding of papilledema, but not all of them. Patients usually consult their doctors because of headaches or neck pain. Sometimes they complain of ringing in the ears, double vision, decreased vision, or odd, very transient episodes of obscured vision. Some will also have nausea and vomiting.

The diagnostic criteria for pseudotumor cerebri include symptoms or signs of elevated intracranial pressure, a normal CT scan (or other brain imaging study), normal spinal fluid (other than the pressure being raised), and a normal physical examination (other than some of the eye findings, most notably papilledema). In some definitions, the doctor must have excluded a clot in the veins of the brain, which can sometimes mimic pseudotumor (an association first described by Nonne). Overall, pseudotumor is a rare condition, and many doctors will go through a career seeing only one or two cases. In children it is even less common than in adults. But it is an important diagnosis to make, because the major complication is that it can lead to permanent blindness if untreated. Various treatments, both medical and surgical, exist.

The pattern of patients in which pseudotumor cerebri appears is curious. It is most commonly seen in overweight adult women, typically in the twenty-to-forty age range. In fact, women are affected nearly ten times more frequently than men, and adults are affected much more commonly than children. In children, though, it is seen equally in boys and girls. In all populations, however, the disease is quite rare. In any population, one thing is clear: doctors do not know why it happens. In cases where the patient does not fit the usual epidemiological pattern (obese adult women), there is a long list of conditions that are associated with the development of pseudotumor, but the nature of what causes it is still unknown, even in these cases.

One of these associated conditions is Lyme disease. This is especially true in North American children with Lyme disease, which is common in the northeast. Pseudotumor cerebri is also associated with various antibiotics especially in the tetracycline group, and with vitamin toxicity, especially vitamin A. Other medications, such as lithium, steroids, oral contraceptives, and hormone replacement therapy, have also been reported to be associated with pseudotumor. Still other cases have been described in patients with abnormal thyroid function, Addison's disease (underactive adrenal glands), lupus, severe anemia, and even cancers. In these instances, simply treating the associated condition will resolve the pseudotumor cerebri.

"So now we had to find the cause of the pseudotumor," Urion said, shaking his head as he recalls how they made the ultimate diagnosis. "We went back and re-asked about medications. Did she take any meds? Did she have access to other peoples' medicines in the house? The family took a little umbrage at our repeated questions. Finally the family asked us, 'What can cause this?' We gave them the list and one of the things on the list is vitamins. They seemed to stop at 'vitamins' on that list. They asked, 'Could fish oil have these vitamins in them?'"

Fish oils, such as cod liver oil, are nutritional supplements made from the fish parts, particularly livers, containing high levels of omega-3 fatty acids and vitamins A and D. Vitamin A, or retinol, is an important substance for normal vision, bone health, neurological development, and various immune functions. As with all vitamins, the U.S. government sets a recommended daily dose, which in the case of vitamin A is expressed as "retinol activity equivalents" (RAE). The daily RAE is a function of age and sex. For a girl of Luisa's age, the daily dose is about 1,350 RAE. Most Americans get enough retinol from the diet. A single carrot, for example, which gets its orange color from a pigment called carotene, has over 1,000 RAE by itself. Other orange foods, such as pumpkin, butternut squash, and sweet potatoes, are also high in vitamin A. Cod liver oil contains about 1,350 RAE per teaspoon.

The next day, the grandmother brought in a bottle of Smith's Fish Emulsion, which contained 100 percent of the adult daily requirement of vitamins A and D in each tablespoon. The directions on the bottle were to take one tablespoon per day, which is what the grandmother dutifully had been giving Luisa. Every other month, for more than a year, this five-year-old child had been getting the recommended daily dose—for an adult—of these vitamins. The vitamin A in the fish oil, of course, was in addition to all that she got in her normal diet.

The oil itself was in some ways a by-product of the North American Free Trade Agreement, which greatly freed up import restrictions, leaving the U.S. pharmaceutical industry manufacturing too much of vitamins A and D for domestic use, and therefore in search of a market for the surplus. It found one in Latin America, where it turned out there was demand for "high-grade," U.S.-approved, pharmaceutical-quality vitamins sold over the counter. Eventually these came to be established products for Latin American consumers, and they started to be sold in Latino bodegas back in North America, which is where Luisa's grandmother found them.

As often happens in unusual cases, there were precedents in the medical literature. One of the first was the remarkable tale of Douglas Mawson and his fellow explorers of Antarctica. In November 1912, Mawson, Belgrave Ninnis, and Xavier Merz set out to map the area near the South Pole. On December 14, disaster struck: Ninnis, along with a husky-pulled sled carrying most of their food, fell to his death in a crevasse. Merz and Mawson had to find their way back to the base camp with extremely low rations, and they ended up killing the remaining sled dogs and eating them. They ate not only the meat, but their livers. Merz died on the return, on January 8, 1913. A full month later, remarkably, Mawson crawled back into camp, on February 8. Several who have studied the expedition believe that Merz and Mawson suffered from vitamin A toxicity from the dog livers. Merz and Ninnis are remembered by having two of the large glaciers in Antarctica named in their honor.

Because vitamin A is fat-soluble, large amounts accumulate in the liver, and other pseudotumor cases have been described in people eating too much liver from bear, shark, seal, and cow. Even carrots have been associated with pseudotumor. In one twenty-seven-year-old obese woman with pseudotumor, her symptoms were resolving with a very successful weight-loss program. After about six months, however, her eyes began to once again show signs of papilledema, even though she continued to successfully lose weight. It turned out she had been eating two to three pounds of raw carrots a week for sixteen months. Vitamin A toxicity was diagnosed when her serum retinol was measured at twice the normal value. Eliminating the carrots from her diet cured the problem, and all the findings resolved.

Vitamin A toxicity has been reported with children eating too many vitamins as well. Because the vitamins are flavored and taste good to children, sometimes they eat them like candy. In patients who have pseudotumor cerebri, blood levels of vitamin A have been found to be elevated, although the mechanism and significance of this finding are not clear.

The best treatment for pseudotumor is not known, partly because the disease is sufficiently uncommon that large well-controlled studies are difficult to organize and perform. If an inciting factor is found—such as the fish oil in Luisa's case—it is eliminated, but often, this is not enough. Some patients are left with permanent visual loss. In patients whose disease is associated with obesity, weight loss is important. Repeated lumbar puncture is another treatment, to reduce the pressure on the optic nerves. Another is a medication called acetazolamide, which is a kind of diuretic used to reduce intraocular pressure. Other diuretics are sometimes used as well.

There are also surgical treatments, the most common being a shunt procedure. In this operation, a neurosurgeon inserts a tube with a one-way pressure valve into the subarachnoid space and diverts the spinal fluid into another part of the body, usually the abdominal cavity, where the fluid is reabsorbed into the bloodstream. The pressure valve can be set at a safe level, and if the spinal fluid pressure rises above that number, the valve opens and the fluid is diverted away from the brain and into the abdominal cavity. The last surgical procedure is an optic nerve fenestration. In this operation, an ophthalmologist makes an incision in the membrane that surrounds the optic nerve. It is not clear why this helps, but in many cases it does.

Most patients with pseudotumor cerebri fully recover, but about 10 percent are left blind in one eye, and nearly half will have some decreased vision.

As Urion sits back in his chair, thinking over Luisa's case in hindsight, he muses, "What it taught me is this. Four of us, all good doctors, had asked about medication ingestion. But none of us asked the question the right way. The family finally helped us out by asking us directly, 'what are you worried about?' That helped us to be more direct with our questions and get to the right answer. My lapsing into medical jargon could have affected the care of the patient. Now I ask the question differently, and I learn more about the patients. In the past, when I asked about medications, I'd often hear nothing, either because the patients were embarrassed that they were taking something that had not been prescribed, or just because they didn't consider some things 'medications,' such as herbs or other nutritional supplements."

"As for Luisa, she underwent multiple lumbar punctures to reduce the pressure; this only worked partially, so we added acetazolamide, which also worked only partially. Then we added furosemide [another diuretic]. She recovered some of her vision, but not completely, and still has occasional headaches." But the problem was diagnosed, at least, and any further loss of vision was halted.

~~~~~~~~~~~~~~~~~~~

Virginia Palazzo, an internist who lives in Belmont, Massachusetts, wasn't the kind of mother who worried over every little thing. But she became very concerned in the spring of 1991 when her eighteen-month-old daughter, Christa, suddenly lost her appetite. The odd thing was that, at the same time, she seemed to be drinking all the fluids she could get. Palazzo also noticed that her daughter wasn't gaining any weight. The situation was even more disturbing when the little girl's pediatrician could not find anything wrong.

"We couldn't figure it out. As an afterthought, the pediatrician checked her blood calcium level."

Meanwhile, in nearby Watertown, Massachusetts, cardiac nurse Lou Goldberg, fifty-eight, wasn't feeling well either. "At first I thought it was all the night shifts or maybe my diabetes," she recalls, even though she had been working nights for years and her diabetes was under good control. Her symptoms were as vague as their onset was insidious—fatigue, nausea, abdominal cramps. "Then I began to lose weight," she says. "I was almost glad, because I'm short and overweight."

But by mid-June, Lou's deteriorating physical condition convinced her to have blood tests. "People would say 'you look awful,' and co-workers knew I was sick and kept urging me to see a doctor. I really didn't feel well; I felt nauseous all the time."

That's when she got scared and went to see her doctor. He drew blood and sent it off for a fairly standard battery of tests—things like a red and white cell count, sodium and potassium, kidney and liver function tests, and of course a blood sugar. Years ago, doctors would have ordered specific tests, but for at least the past couple of decades many are grouped together as a panel of multiple tests. Partly this is due to the equipment; an automated machine can run dozens of tests on a tiny sample of blood just as quickly (if not quicker) as running a single test on an older machine. One of the tests that is a component of these standard panels is the serum calcium. So Goldberg had that checked too. That result, and that one only, came back as quite a surprise. The results showed hypercalcemia—an alarmingly high level of calcium in the blood.

Reduced to its most basic core, and with the water taken away, the human body is simply a pile of chemicals. Roughly two-thirds of the body's weight is water, a bit more if you are a man and a little less if you are a woman. For that reason, oxygen and hydrogen are important chemical components, as are carbon and nitrogen. Because of the large quantity of bones, calcium is the next most common chemical component by weight. Sodium, potassium, phosphorus, sulfur, chlorine, magnesium, iodine, and iron are all present in very small but absolutely critical amounts. Without iron, for example, which makes up about one-tenth of 1 percent of a person's body weight, our red blood cells could not carry oxygen. And certain trace elements such as chromium, copper, and zinc are present in even smaller amounts in the body. But each has its purpose, and without some of these chemical components in the body, we would die.

One could make a shopping list and buy all of these chemicals, and add water. With the right ingredient list and recipe, one could precisely duplicate the concentrations of each of these substances. But of course, we would not have built a human body, a functioning living creature; we would simply have a pile of wet chemicals.

Science fiction aside, no scientist knows the secret that breathes life into this laboratory experiment. Over the past century and a half, though, scientists and physicians have worked out at least some of the more superficial truths. One of the first was Claude Bernard, a Frenchman who is known as the father of physiology. Bernard was born in 1813, and started out dabbling as a writer of vaudeville and theater, but thankfully for humankind, the critics dissuaded him and he ended up in medicine, studying in Paris. Around 1850, Bernard became the inaugural chairman of the physiology department at the Sorbonne. The department lacked a laboratory, but Louis-Napoléon, emperor of France, corrected this deficiency in 1864 and had one built at the National Museum of Natural History.

One of Bernard's major accomplishments was his *Introduction to the Study of Experimental Medicine*, published in 1865. He was one of the first scientists to use the scientific method in a rigorous way. "When we meet a fact which contradicts a prevailing theory, we must accept the fact and abandon the theory, even when the theory is supported by great names and generally accepted," he wrote.

Bernard worked on the effects of various poisons, the importance of the pancreas in digestion, and the role of the liver in maintaining proper levels of glucose in the body. It is this last concept that has an impact on our story. Bernard wrote, "The maintenance of a constant internal environment is the condition for a free and independent life."

In this one sentence, Bernard expressed the physiological concept of what we now call homeostasis. That term, from the Greek *homeo* (same) and *stasis* (standing), was first coined by Walter B. Cannon.

In his book *The Wisdom of the Body*, published in 1932, Cannon wrote,

> *Organisms, composed of material which is characterized by the utmost inconstancy and unsteadiness, have somehow learned the methods of maintaining constancy and keeping steady in the presence of conditions which might reasonably be expected to prove profoundly disturbing. For a short time men may be exposed to dry heat at 115 to 128 degrees Centigrade (239 to 261 degrees Fahrenheit) without an increase of their body temperature above normal. On the other hand arctic mammals, when exposed to cold as low as 35 degrees Centigrade below freezing (31 degrees below zero Fahrenheit) do not manifest any noteworthy fall of body temperature. Furthermore, in regions where the air is extremely dry the inhabitants have little difficulty in retaining their body fluids. And in these days of high ventures in mountain climbing and in airplanes, human beings may be surrounded by a greatly reduced pressure of oxygen in the air without showing serious effects of oxygen want.*

Using Bernard's notions as a foundation, Cannon further developed the concept of homeostasis and described its four basic propositions. To paraphrase, he thought that, first, there must be physiological mechanisms that act to maintain the constancy of the internal environment. He used such examples as glucose concentrations, body temperature, and acid-base balance. Second, he said that there must be a balance of factors that act to change a given state with others that counterbalance the change. Dehydration leads to high serum sodium, which stimulates thirst; drinking water to quench the thirst then corrects the dehydration. His third principle is that the regulation of homeostasis consists of a number of cooperating mechanisms acting simultaneously or successively. If the blood sugar rises, insulin will reduce it back to the normal range; if it falls, other hormones tell the liver to release stored sugar to raise it. And last, homeostasis is not some haphazard or chance event; it requires organization by the body.

Consider the example of homeostasis with regard to serum sodium and potassium levels. There are different compartments in the body: the intracellular compartment (inside of cells), where the potassium concentration is high and the sodium is low; and the extracellular compartment (outside of cells), where just the opposite occurs. Consistent with Cannon's theory, the physiological mechanism that "maintains the constancy of the environment" is an active energy-dependent pump located in the cell membrane that pumps potassium into the cell and sodium out.

Mechanisms are in place to ensure that the blood glucose doesn't go too high or too low. Body temperature is regulated to stay within a very narrow range. The acidity of the body's fluids is also tightly regulated.

One other substance that the body maintains within a very narrow range is the serum calcium.

Although women are constantly urged to get enough calcium to prevent the bone deterioration of osteoporosis, Lou's diagnosis of hypercalcemia was anything but good news. Excess calcium in the blood can eventually become deposited in tissues and organs, causing them to calcify, or harden; what's more, the condition can be a sign of various diseases, including cancer.

Hypercalcemia often announces its presence in a variety of subtle ways, as our two cases illustrate—fatigue, decreased appetite, weight loss, nausea and vomiting, stomach pains, increased urination, constipation, and depression. Mildly elevated levels often produce absolutely no symptoms whatsoever. The condition is often discovered only accidentally when a routine blood panel that includes calcium is checked. However, once identified, hypercalcemia should never be ignored; it's always a sign of an underlying medical problem.

The most common cause of a high blood calcium level is an over-active parathyroid gland, usually resulting from a benign tumor, called an adenoma. If the adenoma pumps out too much parathyroid hormone, or PTH, the action of this hormone causes the body to mobilize calcium from the bone, and the calcium level in the blood can skyrocket.

The second most common cause, especially in older people, is cancer. The cancer can originate from the breast, prostate, kidney, or lung, as well as other parts of the body. These malignancies are often metastatic and often cause other symptoms that are noticed first—back pain from a tumor in the spine, or headache from a brain metastasis, but sometimes hypercalcemia is the earliest and only clue. Together, overactive parathyroid glands and cancer account for nearly 90 percent of cases of hypercalcemia.

Lou Goldberg remembers being frightened. "I was worried about what was causing the high calcium. At first, I didn't want to pursue a work-up. I figured, 'this too shall pass.' But for the first time in my life, I was a little scared. I am not one of those people who, when they get a headache, are worried that it's a brain tumor. I go 100 percent the opposite way, but this time I was worried."

Fortunately, Lou tested negative for both of these two possible problems, leaving her physician baffled. What the doctor didn't know yet was that an alarming number of similar cases were popping up all over the Boston metropolitan area. As it turned out, the cases of eighteen-month-old Christa Palazzo and fifty-eight-year-old Lou Goldberg were strangely linked.

The reports of this phenomenon, scattered at first, began to surface on the desk of Michael Holick, M.D., Ph.D., a nationally renowned expert in vitamin D and calcium metabolism at Boston University School of Medicine. As time went on, more information became available. Like Lou Goldberg, when these other patients had PTH levels drawn, they were always normal; and when tests for cancer were done, they were always negative. But remember that these two problems cause only 90 percent of the cases of hypercalcemia. There are others. Of the first eight cases that Dr. Holick knew about, two came to light when they were independently presented at a Boston inter-hospital joint endocrine conference. Both had unexplained vitamin D intoxication. Six others became known because they were ultimately referred to one of the endocrinologists who had attended that meeting.

Some of the cases were in adults and others were children. This made it unlikely to be a result of parathyroid problems or tumors. Some of the referring physicians checked for, and ruled out, these other causes. The reports that were sent to Holick showed that the patients all had elevated levels of vitamin D as well as calcium. That was the link. Excess vitamin D is another, though considerably less common, cause of hypercalcemia. But why?

A vitamin is an organic substance that is required by the body, usually in extremely small quantities, for the normal function of some metabolic pathway. Until relatively recently in human history, a person's diet was the sole source of vitamins; there were, of course, no supplements. By accumulated experience, doctors learned about the importance of vitamins, usually due to natural experiments of privation. Thus the ancient Egyptians learned that eating liver (high in vitamin A) could cure blindness. The eighteenth-century Scottish physician James Lind observed that a malady sailors in the Royal Navy commonly suffered from, scurvy, could be prevented by eating citrus fruits (hence the term "limeys").

The word "vitamin" comes from the Polish biochemist Kazimierz Funk, who thought that these chemicals were derived from ammonia, or "amines," and were thus "vital amines." The "e" was dropped when it was later found that these chemicals were not amines at all, but the word stuck.

Rickets is a disease that has been known since antiquity. The origin of the name is unknown, but the Greek word *rachitis*, meaning inflammation of the spine, was sufficiently close that scientists used it to mean rickets. The disease is a softening of the bones that results in frequent fractures and severe deformity, most commonly in children. The first clear descriptions date back to 1650 in England. Although the cause was unknown at the time, the disease was quite common. Little progress occurred for nearly two hundred years.

By the late 1800s, rickets was endemic, especially in infants living in northern cities in both the United States and Europe. Theories, but not hard facts, abounded as to its cause. Was it dietary? Or related to poor hygiene? Did it have to do with lack of exercise or of sunlight? In 1889, British scientist John Bland-Sutton showed that lion cubs at the London Zoo, which were fed a diet exclusively of boneless red meat, were developing severe rickets. He found that he could cure the cubs by adding crushed bones and cod liver oil to their feed.

The English physician Edward Mellanby clearly established that diet could play a role in rickets in 1919. American nutritionist Elmer McCollum began a long series of experiments in 1922 that culminated in the discovery of a substance found in the diet that could prevent rickets. It seemed related to, but clearly distinct from, vitamin A. Because the nomenclature for the vitamins followed alphabetical order, A, B, and C had been discovered, so McCollum called this new substance vitamin D.

One thing was clear: cod liver oil, which contained vitamin D, could cure rickets.

But this was only one part of the puzzle. Rickets seemed to be more common in the winter, and occurred more frequently in northern latitudes than in the tropics. Dark-skinned babies were affected more often than light-skinned ones. None of these facts could be explained by a simple dietary deficiency. Some researchers suggested that the seasonality of rickets had to do with the amount of sunlight the children were exposed to. In a series of carefully controlled experiments carried out in Vienna after World War I, Dr. Harriet Chick demonstrated with certainty that exposure to sunlight could prevent or treat rickets.

Later it was shown that not only sunlight but also ultraviolet radiation was sufficient to cure rickets. Later in the last century many experiments done by several groups across the world would show that vitamin D could be produced in the skin by UV light activating a chemical in the skin. The common denominator for rickets was too little vitamin D, whether by a dietary deficiency, insufficient sunlight, or both.

In 1930, as a result of these findings, dairies in the United States began fortifying milk with vitamin D. That single public health intervention dramatically reduced the incidence of rickets, so that the disease is now exceedingly rare in the United States.

But as with almost everything else in life, one can have too much of a good thing.

So now, Holick had to unravel the second part of the puzzle: what was responsible for the high levels of vitamin D? There were only a few possibilities: excessive sunlight, too much vitamin D in the diet (perhaps from cod liver oil or eating lots of fatty fish), or megadose vitamin supplements. He eliminated the excessive sunlight hypothesis immediately —these cases were occurring in New England, and even lifeguards in the tropics almost never develop high vitamin D levels from sunlight alone.

Holick and his colleagues sent out detailed questionnaires to the first eight patients that were identified. "And bingo," recalls Holick, "all of them drank a lot of milk." The last piece of the puzzle now fell neatly and (for these kinds of investigations) rapidly into place. Not only did these patients drink a lot of milk, but they all got their milk from the same dairy, Crescent Ridge, in Sharon, Massachusetts, a small family-run business serving roughly eleven thousand customers in twenty-eight towns in the Boston metropolitan area.

At this point, the Massachusetts Department of Public Health launched a full-scale investigation. But first it ordered Crescent Ridge to stop adding vitamin D to its products. On July 3, 1991, the department sent a notice to area physicians, local boards of health, and customers of Crescent Ridge. It suggested that anyone who had drunk any milk from the dairy since January 1991 have blood tests for calcium and vitamin D levels. The letter read:

> It has come to our attention that an excess amount of vitamin D was added to some milk [products] at the Crescent Ridge Dairy. The dairy has been cooperative and has participated in our efforts to solve this problem. Vitamin D is an optional supplement for milk and the dairy has stopped adding it to its milk since the problem was discovered. . . .
>
> Because the symptoms are vague, we are advising that anyone who has been drinking milk from the Crescent Ridge Dairy since January 1, 1991, should contact their health provider to have blood tests done for calcium. Please bring this notice to your heath care provider. If your calcium is elevated, further medical evaluation will be needed.

The local media quickly picked up the story, and area labs were inundated with requests for blood work. At the Newton Wellesley Hospital, which serves many of the communities where the dairy delivered its products, the lab was inundated. The lab manager said, "Whole families were coming in with the letters [from the public health department]. Many people were quite anxious. We normally will draw blood from about 100 outpatients per day, and over that July Fourth weekend, we were doing 250 and more. Even people who weren't customers of that dairy were asking to have their blood drawn." Of the 1,000 patients tested over a two-week period, only 15 had elevated blood calcium levels; at another nearby hospital, 4 of 630 tested were positive.

Federal regulations state that one quart of milk should contain four hundred international units (ten micrograms) of vitamin D. Toxicity from too much vitamin D is quite rare, but it does happen. The members of one Scottish family fell ill just before Christmas of 1981. The two parents and four children all developed nausea, vomiting, and excessive thirst. The three eldest children, who were boys, were most severely affected; the eleven-year-old needed to be hospitalized first, initially with a diagnosis of "food poisoning." His two brothers needed to be hospitalized over the next forty-eight hours. Doctors found it odd that although they were all dehydrated, their blood pressures were elevated, not low.

Then the doctors found that each one had a severely elevated serum calcium level. So did their seventeen-month-old sister and both parents. Their PTH levels were low, and their vitamin D was high. Something at the house was poisoning them with vitamin D. The levels of calcium fell rapidly, but it took months for the vitamin D levels to fall, partly because it is a fat-soluble vitamin (which helps explain why sun exposure during the summer helps keep the vitamin levels elevated for several months into the fall and winter). The father's peak vitamin D level was 1,287 nanograms per milliliter, almost 25 times higher than the top normal of 50. Despite a thorough search of the house, the public health authorities never found the causative food.

In another case, a healthy two-year-old Hispanic child was seen in an emergency room for constipation and abdominal pain. He was released after a normal physical examination, although the blood pressure was slightly elevated. His mother brought him back the next day for continued symptoms. Again, except for an elevated blood pressure, his exam was normal, but this time the doctor sent blood work. The boy's calcium was elevated, at 14.4 milligrams per deciliter.

On taking the boy's history, the doctors found that his mother was giving him a vitamin D supplement called Raquiferol, normally sold in Latin America but available in bodegas in the United States as well. The recommended dosage was two drops (from an ampoule) per day, but the mother had given the boy a full ampoule each day for four days in a row. Each ampoule contained 600,000 international units (IU). The adequate intake for toddlers is about 200 IU per day; the boy had received 3,000 times the recommended amount. He was severely vitamin D toxic and severely hypercalcemic. After two weeks in the hospital he improved, and fortunately he suffered no lasting effects.

In another bizarre case, a one-year-old dog, a nineteen-pound pug, became toxic from his owner's medication. The owner used a vitamin D analog called calcipotriene cream to treat his psoriasis. The dog was used to licking the owner's skin, and apparently liked the taste of the medicated cream. One day when the medication was inadvertently left unattended, the dog consumed the remainder of a tube of the medicine. Within forty-eight hours, the dog started to vomit blood and seemed unusually fatigued. Despite treatment, the dog died of severe hypercalcemia.

When Holick and the other investigators tested the milk, their results were nothing less than astonishing. Crescent Ridge's homogenized whole milk sold in April 1991 had a vitamin D level of 232,565 IU per quart—nearly 600 times the acceptable amount. Milk from two months later, however, in June, had nearly undetectable amounts. The non-fat and low-fat milk also had levels of vitamin D that were between 75 to 150 times higher than recommended.

Authorities are still not sure precisely how this happened. The concentrate of vitamin D that the dairy employees added to the milk was vitamin D2, labeled as containing 400,000 IU per milliliter. But when Holick had the concentrate tested, it gave results as if it were vitamin D3. Initially, this finding nearly threw the investigators off track. Either the lab was not doing the test correctly, or the dairy was wrong about its D2. But another possibility was that it was not the dairy's fault at all.

Holick was convinced that the source of the problem had to be the dairy. Finally, after repeated testing, he proved that the additive was actually D3, a finding he confirmed by having it submitted to mass spectrophotometry at the National Institutes of Health. The manufacturer, Freeman Industries in New York, had been mislabeling the product. In terms of toxicity, the mislabeling was not a major issue, although vitamin D3 is about three times stronger than D2, so the effects of this error were compounded. More important was that it delayed the investigation by a few months.

On top of everything else, the highly concentrated vitamin solution was being added to the milk by hand at Crescent Ridge (as it is at half the dairies in the country); the investigators speculated that the extreme dosage could have simply been a result of human error.

At last the mysterious symptoms began to make sense for Virginia Palazzo and Lou Goldberg, both of whom were Crescent Ridge customers.

"I was worried that my kids would suffer growth problems or kidney damage," Virginia says. Luckily, that did not occur. "It wasn't easy keeping an eight-year-old and an eighteen-month-old out of the sun or covered up with sunscreen all summer, but you do your best," says Palazzo.

Lou Goldberg was relieved as well. "I can't drink a lot of sweet sodas and juices because of my diabetes," she explains. "And because I am allergic to aspartame, diet sodas are out, and I don't like coffee or tea. So I've always enjoyed milk. I drink loads of it. Some people are alcoholics; I drink a lot of milk, but I had to decrease my milk intake, so I did."

It's not known exactly how many people experienced symptoms of hypercalcemia, but the number was likely low given how few patients who were tested actually had elevated calcium levels.

The incident at Crescent Ridge sparked calls for a reevaluation of milk processing and inspection nationwide.

Soon afterward, Holick checked out other brands of milk, buying forty-two samples from various dairies and supermarkets in five eastern states. The first results of his investigation, published in the *New England Journal of Medicine*, were unsettling. Out of all forty-two containers labeled "vitamin-D fortified," 80 percent fell outside the acceptable range. Sixty-two percent of those quarts contained too little vitamin D (some had none at all), which could be harmful for youngsters or older women, many of whom depend on milk for their daily requirements.

The remainder had too much vitamin D (though none had levels as high as Crescent Ridge's).

He also tested infant formula from five major national suppliers. All contained more than 150 percent of the amount of vitamin D stated on the label. While no life-threatening overdoses were found, the study demonstrates how easily an error could go undetected.

It's not mandatory that vitamin D be added to milk, but most dairies do fortify their product. Those that do are required to state it on the label. The mandated amount is 400 IUs per quart, but regulations permit a 140 percent margin of error.

Monitoring of vitamin D levels and other safety issues, such as bacterial contamination, is under the control of the FDA if the milk is sold across state lines. Small dairies like Crescent Ridge, which sell their milk in only one state, are not under federal jurisdiction, but they are supposed to test their milk twice a year to be sure that the amount of vitamin D falls within the range stipulated by the FDA.

Budget cuts have affected the FDA's ability to properly inspect milk. In response to the outbreak, an article in the *Boston Globe* on July 21, 1991, reported:

> *The FDA has only 23 people assigned to milk safety nationwide, down from 33 a decade ago. The job of overseeing the system in New England has changed hands five times in the last eight years. The last person to hold it left last week. The federal agency is responsible for close to 1000 dairies and 150,000 farms.*
>
> *Budget-strapped state governments, which share responsibility with the FDA, are cutting their milk inspection staffs. In the past two years, the New England states have sliced the number of inspectors by more than a third to 35. According to the FDA, four of the six states do not perform the test that would have caught the problem at [Crescent Ridge] even though federal rules require it be done.*

In the same article, the director of the Massachusetts Department of Public Health's food and drug division said of that test, "We haven't done it in years. We don't have the [personnel]."

Despite this outbreak of vitamin D toxicity, the vitamin's use in milk is important. In Britain, in 1956, the British Pediatric Society found that 204 cases of hypercalcemia from vitamin D intoxication had occurred over a two-year period. This resulted in the cessation of the vitamin D milk fortification program in Great Britain. But when the incidence of rickets shot up as a result, the experiment was quickly abandoned. Nevertheless, these cases show that, as with all beneficiary interventions, they must be implemented wisely and cautiously.

All that said, the Crescent Ridge case clearly illustrates the potential toxic effects of excessive vitamin D. Holick and other experts urge that dairies use advanced measurement and quality-control techniques and that regulatory agencies enforce guidelines by routinely analyzing the vitamin D content of fortified foods. Even simple quality assurance measures would have shown a serious problem. Had the dairy been using the supplement correctly, it should have been using less than three bottles of the vitamin concentrate each year. But according to Massachusetts officials, Crescent Ridge used fifty-five bottles in 1989 and eighty-five bottles in 1990.

In the Crescent Ridge outbreak, the first case that was identified occurred roughly a year before the last one, and the dairy had been adding too much vitamin D in its milk for two years before the outbreak surfaced. Putting this together was in part fortuitous but in part related to the cooperative spirit of Boston's doctors. Holick and his co-authors wrote in their medical report of the affair: "This study illustrates the importance of discussing cases that do not appear to have an explanation in a hospital or inter-hospital conference. It is from such a forum that a unifying thread may emerge. The search for a common vehicle in these cases led to a review of each patient's dietary history (with use of a questionnaire) that in no instance revealed the ingestion of an unusual type or amount of food. All patients, however, obtained their milk from the same dairy." Without that conference, it's quite possible that many more people would have become affected and some might have had worse outcomes.

In fact, one seventy-two-year-old woman from Norwood, Massachusetts, had a prolonged hospitalization and died, although the precise contribution of the hypercalcemia is not known. As for Lou Goldberg, she drastically cut down on milk intake, and by August 1991, she was feeling perfectly normal. Similarly, the Palazzo children were also fine in the end. Both the children and Ms. Goldberg had follow-up calcium levels that were normal, and fortunately none of them seemed to have any long-lasting effects.

Sources

~~~~~~

Some of the pieces in this book were previously published in shorter forms and, in some cases, under different titles. The chapters that first appeared in *Boston Magazine* are "A Study in Scarlet" (June 1989, under the title "Something Fishy"), "An Airtight Case" (September 1989), "Feeling His Oats" (January 1990), "The Case of the Wide-Eyed Boy" (May 1990), and "The Case of the Overly Hot Honeymoon" (October 1990, under the title "The Woman Who Ate Too Much"). Those that appeared in *Ladies' Home Journal* are "The Deadly Dinner Party" (May 1990, under the title "The Case of the Deadly Dinner Party"), "The Baby and the Bathwater" (February 1991, under the title "The Case of the Careful Babysitter"), "Too Much of a Good Thing" (September 1992), "The Case of the Unhealthy Health Food" (February 1993), "The Forbidden Fruit" (October 1994, under the title "The Case of the Fallen Fruit"), and "Rubbed the Wrong Way" (November 1994, under the title "The Case of the Peculiar Pimples").

Chapter 1. The Deadly Dinner Party

"Botulism Poisoning Case Prompts Garlic-Oil Warning." *Kingston (N.Y.) Freeman*, March 1, 1989.

Burros, Marian. "Eating Well." *New York Times*, May 3, 1989.

Centers for Disease Control and Prevention (CDC). "Botulism from Fresh Foods: California." *Morbidity and Mortality Weekly Report (MMWR)* 34 (1985): 156–57.

Centers for Disease Control and Prevention (CDC). "International Outbreak of Type E Botulism Associated with Ungutted, Salted Whitefish." *Morbidity and Mortality Weekly Report (MMWR)* 36 (1987): 812–13.

Centers for Disease Control and Prevention (CDC). "Type B Botulism Associated with Roasted Eggplant in Oil: Italy 1993." *Morbidity and Mortality Weekly Report (MMWR)* 44 (1995): 33–36.

Centers for Disease Control and Prevention (CDC). "Wound Botulism Among Black Tar Heroin Users—Washington 2003." *Morbidity and Mortality Weekly Report (MMWR)* 52 (2003): 885–86.

Charnow, Jody. "Stricken Trio Beats the Odds." *Kingston (N.Y.) Freeman*, February 28, 1989.

Christie, A. B., ed. *Infectious Diseases: Epidemiology and Clinical Practice.* 2nd ed. Edinburgh: Churchill Livingstone (1974), chapter 6.

Consumer Affairs. "Castleberry Botulism Recall Expanded." http://www.consumer affairs.com/news04/2007/07/botulism_recall.html (accessed December 2007).

"Death in Cans." *Time Magazine*, July 19, 1971.

Erbguth, F. J. "From Poison to Remedy: The Chequered History of Botulinum Toxin." *Journal of Neural Transmission* 4 (2007): 559–65.

Erbguth, F. J., and M. Naumann. "Historical Aspects of Botulinum Toxin: Justinus Kerner (1786–1862) and the 'Sausage Poison.'" *Neurology* 53 (1999): 1850–53.

"FDA Issues Botulism Warning." *Kingston (N.Y.) Freeman*, March 7, 1989.

Food Poison Blog. "Castleberry's Botulism Outbreak Update." http://www.food poisonblog.com/2007/10/articles/foodborne-illness-outbreaks/castleberrys-botulism-outbreak-update.html (accessed December 2007).

Horwitz, M. A., J. M. Hughes, M. H. Merson, and E. J. Gangarosa. "Food-Borne Botulism in the United States, 1970–1975." *Journal of Infectious Diseases* 136 (1977): 153–59.

Hougherty, Gary A., and Charles A. Kaysner. "Incidence of *Clostridium botulinum* Type E in Alaskan Salmon." *Applied Microbiology* 18 (1980): 950–51.

Hughes, J. M., et al. "Clinical Features of Types A and B Food-Borne Botulism." *Annals of Internal Medicine* 95 (1981): 442–45.

Jankovic, J., and M. F. Brin. "Therapeutic Uses of Botulism Toxin." *New England Journal of Medicine* 324 (1991): 1186–94.

MacDonald, K. L., et al. "Type A Botulism From Sautéed Onions." *Journal of the American Medical Association* 253 (1985): 1275–78.

New York State Department of Public Health. Food-Borne Illness Summary Report. February 21, 1989. Investigator: Brian Devine of the Ulster County Health Department.

Reynolds, Hugh. "Mario: Get off SUNY's Case." *Times Herald-Record* (Middletown, N.Y.), March 5, 1989.

Reynolds, Hugh. "Party Conflict in Kingston." *Times Herald-Record* (Middletown, N.Y.), March 15, 1989.

Reynolds, Hugh. "Some Food for Thought." *Times Herald-Record* (Middletown, N.Y.), March 1, 1989.

St. Louis, M. E., et al., "Botulism from Chopped Garlic: Delayed Recognition of a Major Outbreak." *Annals of Internal Medicine* 108 (1988): 363–67.

Souayah, N., et al. "Severe Botulism After Focal Injection of Botulinum Toxin." *Neurology* 67 (2006): 1855–56.

State of Alaska, Department of Health and Social Services. "Botulism in Alaska: A Guide for Physicians and Health Care Providers—1998 Update." http://www .epi.hss.state.ak.us/pubs/botulism/bot_05.htm (accessed November 2007).

Sterba, James P. "The History of Botulism." *New York Times*, April 28, 1982, Health section.

"Three Remain in Intensive Care with Symptoms of Food Poisoning." *Kingston (N.Y.) Freeman*, February 26, 1989.

Chapter 2. Everywhere That Mary Went

"The Aberdeen Typhoid Outbreak." *British Medical Journal* 2(5425) (December 26, 1964): 1652–54.

Birkhead, Guthrie S., et al. "An Outbreak of Typhoid Fever Associated with a Resort Hotel in New York State." (Health) report PA #89–55 (1989): 1–12.

Birkhead, Guthrie S., et al. "Typhoid Fever at a Resort Hotel in New York: A Large

Outbreak with an Unusual Vehicle." *Journal of Infectious Diseases* 167 (1993): 1228–32.

Bollet, Alfred J. "Lessons from Medical History: And Everywhere That Mary Went." *Resident and Staff Physician* 29 (1993): 101–8.

Bonn, D. "Typhoid Carriers Key to Global Transmission." *Lancet Infectious Diseases* 7 (2007): 14–15.

Burns, M. C. "Typhoid Is Traced to Orange Juice." *Syracuse Herald-Journal*, July 25, 1989.

Christie, A. B. *Infectious Diseases: Epidemiology and Clinical Practice*. 2nd ed. Edinburgh: Churchill Livingston (1974), chapter 3, "Typhoid and Paratyphoid Fevers."

Diack, Leslie, and David Smith. "Sensationalism and Secrecy: The Aberdeen Typhoid Outbreak, 1964." *History Scotland Magazine: Scottish History and Archaeology*, http://www.historyscotland.com/features/aberdeentyphoid.html (accessed November 2007).

Dixon, B. "Anderson's Insight into Aberdeen Mystery." *Lancet Infectious Diseases* 6 (2006): 322.

Feldman, R. E., et al. "Epidemiology of *Salmonella typhi* Infection in a Migrant Labor Camp in Dade County, Florida." *Journal of Infectious Diseases* 130 (1974): 334–42.

Gonzalez-Cortes, A., et al. "Bottled Beverages and Typhoid Fever: The Mexican Epidemic of 1972–1973." *American Journal of Public Health* 72 (1982): 844–45.

Hirsch, Melanie. "County Leads State in Typhoid with Case No. 6." *The Post-Standard* (Syracuse, N.Y.), August 1, 1989.

Hirsch, Melanie. "Eight Develop Symptoms of Typhoid Fever." *The Post-Standard* (Syracuse, N.Y.), July 13, 1989.

Hirsch, Melanie. "Firefighters Bring Typhoid Fever Back From Convention." *The Post-Standard* (Syracuse, N.Y.), July 13, 1989.

Hirsch, Melanie. "Typhoid Fever Spreads in Central New York." *The Post-Standard* (Syracuse, N.Y.), July 14, 1989.

Hoffman, T. A., et al. "Waterborne Typhoid Fever in Dade County, Florida." *American Journal of Medicine* 59 (1975): 481–86.

Leavitt, Judith Walzer. *Typhoid Mary*. Boston: Beacon, 1997.

Mermin, Jonathan H., et al. "Typhoid Fever in the United States: 1985–1994." *Archives of Internal Medicine* 158 (1998): 633–38.

Moorhead, Robert. "William Budd and Typhoid Fever." *Journal of the Royal Society of Medicine* 95 (2002): 561–64.

Nelis, Karen. "Two More Local Cases of Typhoid Diagnosed." *The Post-Standard* (Syracuse, N.Y.), July 25, 1989.

Olsen, J. S., et al. "Outbreaks of Typhoid Fever in the United States, 1960–1999." *Epidemiology of Infections* 130 (2003): 13–21.

Ryan, C. A., N. T. Hargrett-Bean, and P. A. Blake. "*Salmonella typhi* Infections in the United States; 1975–1984." *Review of Infectious Diseases* 11 (1989): 1–8.

Smith, Amber. "First Typhoid Outbreak This Decade." *Syracuse Herald-Journal*, July 20, 1989.

Smith, Amber. "Outbreak of Typhoid Could Be Disastrous." *Syracuse Herald-Journal*, July 13, 1989.

Smith, Amber. "Typhoid Fever in Second Wave of Its Spread." *Syracuse Herald-Journal*, August 1, 1989.

Smith, David. "History and Policy Paper: Lessons for Food Safety Policy from the Aberdeen Typhoid Outbreak in 1964." *History and Policy: Connecting Historians, Policymakers, and the Media,* http://www.historyandpolicy.org/papers/policy-paper-32.html (accessed November 2007).

Taylor, A., A. Santiago, A. Gonzalez-Cortez, and E. J. Gangarosa, et al. "Outbreak of Typhoid Fever in Trinidad in 1971 Tracked to a Commercial Ice Cream Product." *American Journal of Epidemiology* 100 (1974): 150–57.

Taylor, D. N., R. A. Pollard, and P. A. Blake. "Typhoid in the United States and the Risk to the International Traveler." *Journal of Infectious Diseases* 148 (1983): 599–602.

"Two Local Firemen Catch Typhoid Fever at State Convention." *Syracuse Herald-Journal*, July 12, 1989.

Chapter 3. The Baby and the Bathwater

Arai, T., et al. "A Survey of *Plesiomonas shigelloides* from Aquatic Environments, Domestic Animals, Pets, and Humans." *Journal of Hygiene (London)* 84 (1980): 203–11.

Blake, P. A. "Vibrios on the Half Shell: What the Walrus and the Carpenter Didn't Know." *Annals of Internal Medicine* 99 (1983): 558–59.

Blake, P. A., et al. "Cholera—A Possible Endemic Focus in the United States." *New England Journal of Medicine* 302 (1980) 305–9.

Brenden, R. A., M. A. Miller, and J. M. Janda. "Clinical Disease Spectrum and Pathogenic Factors Associated with *Plesiomonas shigelloides* Infections in Humans." *Review of Infectious Diseases* 10 (1988): 303–16.

Centers for Disease Control and Prevention (CDC). "Aquarium-Associated *Plesiomonas shigelloides* Infection—Missouri." *Morbidity and Mortality Weekly Report (MMWR)* 38 (1989): 617–19.

Centers for Disease Control and Prevention (CDC). "Cholera in Louisiana—Update." *Morbidity and Mortality Weekly Report (MMWR)* 35 (1986): 687–88.

Centers for Disease Control and Prevention (CDC). "Toxigenic Vibrio Cholera 01 Infections—Louisiana and Florida." *Morbidity and Mortality Weekly Report (MMWR)* 35 (1986): 606–7.

Chomel, Bruno B. "Zoonoses of House Pets Other than Dogs, Cats, and Birds." *Pediatric Infectious Disease Journal* 11 (1992): 479–87.

Clark, R. B., P. D. Lister, L. Arneson-Rotert, and J. M. Janda. "In vitro Susceptibilities of *Plesiomonas shigelloides* to 24 Antibiotics and Antibiotic Beta-Lactamase Inhibitor Combinations." *Antimicrobial Agents and Chemotherapy* 34 (1990): 159–60.

Davis, W. A. 2nd, J. H. Chretien, V. G. Garagusi, and M. A. Goldstein. "Snake-to-Human Transmission of *Aeromonas shigelloides* Resulting in Gastroenteritis." *Southern Medical Journal* 71 (1978): 474–76.

Fischer, K., et al. "Pseudo-Appendicitis Caused by *Plesiomonas shigelloides*." *Journal of Clinical Microbiology* 26 (1988): 2675–76.

Holmberg, S. D., et al. "*Plesiomonas* Enteric Infections in the United States." *Annals of Internal Medicine* 105 (1986): 690–94.

Ingram, C. W., A. J. Morrison Jr., and R. E. Levit. "Gastroenteritis, Sepsis, and Osteomyelitis Caused by *Plesiomonas shigelloides* in an Immuno-Competent Host: Case Report and Review of the Literature." *Journal of Clinical Microbiology* 25 (1987): 1791–93.

Kain, K. C., and M. T. Kelly. "Antimicrobial Susceptibility of *Plesiomonas shigelloides* from Patients with Diarrhea." *Antimicrobial Agents and Chemotherapy* 33 (1989): 1609–10.

Kain, K. C., and M. T. Kelly. "Clinical Features, Epidemiology, and Treatment of *Plesiomonas shigelloides* Diarrhea." *Journal of Clinical Microbiology* 27 (1998): 998–1001.

Lewbart, Greg. "Ask the Expert." *NOVA Science Now*, http://www.pbs.org/wgbh/nova/sciencenow/3214/04-ask.html (accessed December 2007).

Pathak, Ambadas, Joseph R. Custer, and Josef Levy. "Neonatal Septicemia and Meningitis Due to *Plesiomonas shigelloides*." *Pediatrics* 71 (1983): 389–91.

Paul, R., A. Siitonen, and P. Kèrkkèinen. "*Plesiomonas shigelloides* Bacteremia in a Healthy Girl with Mild Gastroenteritis." *Journal of Clinical Microbiology* 28 (1990): 1455–56.

Pavia, A. T., et al. "Cholera from Raw Oysters Shipped Interstate." *Journal of the American Medical Association* 258 (1987): 2374.

Reinhardt, J. F., and L. George. "*Plesiomonas shigelloides*-Associated Diarrhea." *Journal of the American Medial Association* 253 (1985): 3294–95.

Roth, T., C. Hentsch, P. Erard, and P. Tschantz. "Pyosalpinx: Not Always a Sexually Transmitted Disease? Pyosalpinx Caused by *Plesiomonas shigelloides* in an Immuno-Competent Host." *Clinics in Microbiology and Infection* 8 (2002): 803–5.

Sanyal, D., S. H. Burge, and P. G. Hutchings. "Enteric Pathogens in Tropical Aquaria." *Epidemiology and Infection* 99 (1987): 635–40.

"Two Cases of Continuous Ambulatory Peritoneal Dialysis-Associated Peritonitis Due to *Plesiomonas shigelloides*." *Journal of Clinical Microbiology* 42 (2004): 933–35.

University of Victoria Aquatic Disease Zoonoses Prevention, statement ratified November 2, 2005. http://carc.ucsc.edu/Health%20and%20Safety/Zoonosis/Fish%20Zoonosis.html, http://depts.washington.edu/rubelab/occupational%20health/zoofish.html (accessed December 2007).

Washington State Board of Health. "Zoonotic Diseases and Exotic Pets: A Public Health Policy Assessment." April 2006.

Woo, Patrick C. Y., Susanna K. P. Lau, Samson S. Y. Wong, and Kwok-Yung Yuen. "Zoonotic Disease Potentials of Tropical Fish." http://depts.washington.edu/rubelab/occupational%20health/zoofish.html (accessed December 2007).

Chapter 4. Rubbed the Wrong Way

Agger, D. A., and A. Mardan. "*Pseudomonas aeruginosa* Infections of Intact Skin." *Clinical Infectious Diseases* 20 (1995): 302–8.

Berrouane, Y. F., et al. "Outbreak of Severe *Pseudomonas aeruginosa* Infections

Caused by a Contaminated Drain in a Whirlpool Bathtub." *Clinical Infectious Diseases* 31 (2000): 1331–37.

Bottone, E. J., and A. A. Perez. "*Pseudomonas aeruginosa* Folliculitis Acquired Through Use of a Contaminated Loofah Sponge: An Unrecognized Potential Public Health Problem." *Journal of Clinical Microbiology* 31 (1993): 480–83.

Bottone, E. J., A. A. Perez 2nd, and J. L. Oeser. "Loofah Sponges as Reservoirs and Vehicles in the Transmission of Potentially Pathogenic Bacterial Species to Human Skin." *Journal of Clinical Microbiology* 32 (1994): 469–72.

Bottone, E. J., et al. "Exfoliative Devices: Clandestine Role in the Transmission of Bacterial Pathogens to Human Skin." *Clinical Microbiology Updates* 5(3) (1994): 1–4.

Centers for Disease Control and Prevention (CDC). "An Outbreak of *Pseudomonas* folliculitis Associated with a Waterslide—Utah." *Morbidity and Mortality Weekly Report (MMWR)* 32 (1983): 425–27.

Centers for Disease Control and Prevention (CDC). "*Pseudomonas dermatitis/folliculitis* Associated with Pools and Hot Tubs—Colorado and Maine." *Morbidity and Mortality Weekly Report* 49 (2008): 1087–91.

Crnich, Christopher J., Barbara Gordon, and David Andes. "Hot Tub Associated Necrotizing Pneumonia Due to *Pseudomonas aeruginosa*." *Clinical Infectious Diseases* 36 (2003): e55–57.

Frenkel, L. M. "*Pseudomonas* Folliculitis from Sponges Promoted as Beauty Aids." *Journal of Clinical Microbiology* 31 (1993): 2838–39.

Gustafson, T. L., J. D. Band, R. H. Hutcheson Jr., and W. Schaffner. "*Pseudomonas* Folliculitis: An Outbreak and Review." *Review of Infectious Diseases* 5 (1983): 1–8.

Hewitt, David J., David A. Weeks, Glen C. Milner, and Gail R. Huss. "Industrial *Pseudomonas* Folliculitis." *American Journal of Industrial Medicine* 49 (2006): 895–99.

Highsmith, A. K., P. N. Le, R. F. Khabbaz, and V. P. Munn. "Characteristics of *Pseudomonas aeruginosa* Isolated from Whirlpool and Bathers." *Infection Control* 6 (1985): 407–12.

Hillier, Andrew, Jessica R. Alcorn, Lynette K. Cole, and Joseph Kowalski. "Pyoderma Caused by *Pseudomonas aeruginosa* Infection in Dogs: 20 Cases." *Veterinary Dermatology* 17 (2006): 432–39.

Hoadley, A. W., Gloria Ajello, and Nola Masterson. "Preliminary Studies of Fluorescent Pseudomonas Capable of Growth at 41 Centigrade in Swimming Pool Waters." *Applied Microbiology* 29 (1975): 527–31.

Hoang, T. L. "Culturing Microorganisms from Kitchen Sponges: A Goal to Increased Awareness of Hygiene." Senior independent project, research tutorial HAS 490 (Medical Technology Program, State University of New York at Stony Brook), June 2, 1993.

Jacobson, J. A., A. W. Hoadley, and J. J. Farmer 3rd. "*Pseudomonas aeruginosa* Serogroup 11 and Pool-Associated Skin Rash." *American Journal of Public Health* 66 (1976): 1092.

Kappers, M. H., Johan M. van der Klooster, Rob J. Th Ouwendijk, and Ad Dees. "Community Acquired Necrotizing Fasciitis Due to *Pseudomonas aeruginosa*." *Intensive Care Medicine* 32 (2006): 1093–94.

Kush, B. J., and A. J. Hoadley. "Preliminary Survey of the Association of *Pseudomonas aeruginosa* with Commercial Whirlpool Bath Waters." *American Journal of Public Health* 70 (1980): 279–81.

Maniatis, A. N., et al. "*Pseudomonas aeruginosa* Folliculitis Due to Non-O: 11 Serogroups: Acquisition Through Use of Contaminated Synthetic Sponges." *Clinical Infectious Disease* 21 (1995): 437–39.

Price, D., and D. G. Ahearn. "Incidence and Persistence of *Pseudomonas aeruginosa* in Whirlpools." *Journal of Clinical Microbiology* 26 (1988): 1650–54.

Ratnam, S., K. Hogan, S. B. March, and R. W. Butler. "Whirlpool Associated Folliculitis Caused by *Pseudomonas aeruginosa*: Report of an Outbreak and Review." *Journal of Clinical Microbiology* 23 (1986): 655–59.

Rinke, C. M. "Hot Tub Hygiene." *Journal of the American Medical Association* 250 (1983): 2031.

Rose, H. D., et al. "*Pseudomonas* Pneumonia Associated with Use of a Home Whirlpool Spa." *Journal of the American Medical Association* 250 (1983): 2027–29.

Salmen, P., D. M. Dwyer, H. Vorse, and W. Kruse. "Whirlpool Associated *Pseudomonas aeruginosa* Urinary Tract Infections." *Journal of the American Medical Association* 250 (1983): 2025–26.

Schlech, W. F. 3rd, N. Simonsen, R. Sumarah, and R. S. Martin. "Nosocomial Outbreak of *Pseudomonas aeruginosa* Folliculitis Associated with a Physiotherapy Pool." *Canadian Medical Association Journal* 134 (1986): 909–13.

Scupham, R., et al. "Caribbean Sponge-Related *Pseudomonas* Folliculitis." *Journal of the American Medical Association* 258 (1987): 1608–9.

Sheth, K. J., et al. "*Pseudomonas aeruginosa* Otitis Externa in an Infant Associated with a Contaminated Infant Bath Sponge." *Pediatrics* 77 (1986): 920–21.

Tate, D., S. Mawer, and A. Newton. "Outbreak of *Pseudomonas aeruginosa* Folliculitis Associated with a Swimming Pool Inflatable." *Epidemiology and Infection* 130 (2003): 187–92.

Thomas, P., et al. "*Pseudomonas* Dermatitis Associated with a Swimming Pool." *Journal of the American Medical Association* 253 (1985): 1156–59.

Todar, Kenneth. "*Pseudomonas aeruginosa*." *Todar's Online Textbook of Bacteriology*, http://www.textbookofbacteriology.net/pseudomonas.html (accessed December 2007).

Vog, R., et al. "*Pseudomonas aeruginosa* Skin Infections in Persons Using a Whirlpool in Vermont." *Journal of Clinical Microbiology* 15 (1982): 571–74.

Washburn, J., J. A. Jacobson, E. Marston, and B. Thorsen. "*Pseudomonas aeruginosa* Rash Associated with a Whirlpool." *Journal of the American Medical Association* 235 (1976): 2205–7.

Watts, R. W., and R. A. Dall. "An Outbreak of *Pseudomonas* Folliculitis in Women After Leg Waxing." *Medical Journal of Australia* 144 (1986): 163–64.

Yu, Y., et al., "Hot Tub Folliculitis or Hot Hand-Foot Syndrome Caused by *Pseudomonas aeruginosa*." *Journal of American Academic Dermatology* 57 (2007): 596–600.

Zacherle, B. J., and D. S. Silver. "Hot Tub Folliculitis: A Clinical Syndrome." *Western Journal of Medicine* 137 (1982): 191–94.

Zichini, L. A., Gaetano Asta, and Giuseppe Noto. *Pseudomonas aeruginosa* Folliculitis After Shower/Bath." *International Journal of Dermatology* 39 (2000): 270–73.

Chapter 5. The Forbidden Fruit

Allday, Erin. "*E. Coli* and the Centralization of the Food Industry." *San Francisco Chronicle*, September 23, 2006.

Artis, Joanne Ball. "Word in *E. coli* Case in Rhode Island Is Prevention, not Overreaction." *Boston Globe*, March 22, 1993.

Banatvala, N., et al. "The United States National Prospective Hemolytic Uremic Syndrome Study: Microbiologic, Serologic, Clinical, and Epidemiologic Findings." *Journal of Infectious Diseases* 183 (2001): 1063–70.

Bell, B. P., et al. "A Multi-State Outbreak of *E. coli* O157:H7-Associated Bloody Diarrhea and Hemolytic Uremic Syndrome from Hamburgers: The Washington Experience." *Journal of the American Medical Association* 272 (1994): 1349–53.

Besser, B. E., et al. "An Outbreak of Diarrhea and Hemolytic Uremic Syndrome from *E. coli* O157:H7 in Fresh-Pressed Apple Cider." *Journal of the American Medical Association* 269 (1993): 2217–20.

Blaser, M. J. "Bacteria and Diseases of Unknown Cause: Hemolytic Uremic Syndrome." *Journal of Infectious Diseases* 189 (2004): 552–63.

Boyce, Thomas G., David L. Swerdlow, and Patricia M. Griffin, "*E. coli* O157:H7 and the Hemolytic Uremic Syndrome." *New England Journal of Medicine* 333 (1995): 364–68.

Burros, Marian. "Agriculture Department Policy Blamed for Tainted Food." *New York Times*, March 3, 1993, Health section.

Centers for Disease Control and Prevention (CDC). "Epidemiological Notes and Reports: Thrombotic Thrombocytopenic Purpura Associated with *Escherichia coli* O157:H7." *Morbidity and Mortality Weekly Report (MMWR)* 35 (1986): 549–51.

Centers for Disease Control and Prevention (CDC). "*Escherichia coli* O157:H7 Outbreak Linked to Home-Cooked Hamburgers—California, July 1993." *Morbidity and Mortality Weekly Report (MMWR)* 43 (1994): 213–16.

Centers for Disease Control and Prevention (CDC). "Hemolytic Uremic Syndrome—New York, Massachusetts, Virginia, and District of Columbia." *Morbidity and Mortality Weekly Report (MMWR)* 32 (1983): 578, 584–85.

Centers for Disease Control and Prevention (CDC). "International Notes: Outbreaks of Hemorrhagic Colitis—Ottawa, Canada." *Morbidity and Mortality Weekly Report (MMWR)* 10 (1983): 133–34.

Centers for Disease Control and Prevention (CDC). "Isolation of *Escherichia coli* O157:H7 from Sporadic Cases of Hemorrhagic Colitis—United States." *Morbidity and Mortality Weekly Report (MMWR)* 46 (1982): 700–704.

Centers for Disease Control and Prevention (CDC). "Laboratory Screening for *Escherichia coli* O157:H7—Connecticut, 1993." *Morbidity and Mortality Weekly Report (MMWR)* 43 (1993): 192–94.

Centers for Disease Control and Prevention (CDC). "Lake-Associated Outbreak of

Escherichia coli O157:H7—Illinois, 1995." *Morbidity and Mortality Weekly Report (MMWR)* 45 (1996): 437–39.

Centers for Disease Control and Prevention (CDC). "Outbreak of *Escherichia coli* O157:H7 Infections Associated with Drinking Unpasteurized Commercial Apple Juice—British Columbia, California, Colorado, and Washington, October 1996." *Morbidity and Mortality Weekly Report (MMWR)* 45 (1996): 975.

Centers for Disease Control and Prevention (CDC). "Outbreaks of *Escherichia coli* O157:H7 Associated with Petting Zoos—North Carolina, Florida, and Arizona, 2004 and 2005." *Morbidity and Mortality Weekly Report (MMWR)* 54 (2003): 1277–80.

Centers for Disease Control and Prevention (CDC). "Outbreaks of *Escherichia coli* O157:H7 Infection and Cryptosporidiosis Associated with Drinking Unpasteurized Apple Cider—Connecticut and New York." *Morbidity and Mortality Weekly Report (MMWR)* 46 (1996): 4–8.

Centers for Disease Control and Prevention (CDC). "Preliminary Report: Food Borne Outbreak of *Escherichia coli* O157:H7 Infection from Hamburgers—Western United States, 1993." *Morbidity and Mortality Weekly Report (MMWR)* 42 (1993): 85–86.

Centers for Disease Control and Prevention (CDC). "Update: Multistate Outbreak of *Escherichia coli* O157:H7 Infections from Hamburgers—Western United States, 1992–1993." *Morbidity and Mortality Weekly Report (MMWR)* 42 (1993): 258–63.

Center for Disease Prevention and Epidemiology, Oregon Health Division. "Unpasteurized Juices Strike Again (and Again)." *Current Disease Summary* 45, no. 4 (1996).

Chang, H. H., et al. "Hemolytic Uremic Syndrome Incidence in New York." *Emerging Infectious Diseases* 10 (298): 928–31.

Commonwealth of Massachusetts, Department of Health and Human Services. Public health bulletins, November 29, 1991, January 13, 1992, and the related CDC report dated February 14, 1992.

Davey, Monica. "As Children Suffer, Parents Agonize over Spinach." *New York Times*, September 24, 2006, U.S. section.

Engel, Mary. "*E. coli* Haunts Victims Long After Outbreak." *Los Angeles Times*, September 28, 2006.

Friedman, M. S., et al. "*E. coli* O157:H7-Outbreak Associated With Improperly Chlorinated Swimming Pool." *Clinical Infectious Diseases* 29 (1999): 298–303.

Hillborn, E. D., et al. "An Outbreak of *Escherichia coli* O157:H7 Infection and Hemolytic Uremic Syndrome Associated with Consumption of Unpasteurized Apple Cider." *Epidemiology and Infection* 124 (2000): 31–36.

"Infection Linked to Tainted Cider." *New York Times*, May 6, 1993.

Kolata, Gina. "Detective Work and Science Reveal a New Lethal Bacteria." *New York Times*, January 6, 1998, Health section.

McCarthy, T. A. "Hemolytic Uremic Syndrome and *E. coli* O157:H7 at a Lake in Connecticut—1999." *Pediatrics* 108 (2001): e59–67.

Marler Clark Attorneys at Law, LLP, PS. "Jack in the Box *E. coli* Outbreak—Western States." http://www.marlerclark.com/case_news/view/jack-in-the-box-e-coli-outbreak-western-states (accessed December 2007).

Mello, Michael. "Swansea Cider Linked to Illness." *The Standard-Times* (Fall River, Mass.), January 15, 1992.

Millard, P. S., et al. "An Outbreak of Cryptosporidiosis from Fresh-Pressed Apple Cider." *Journal of the American Medical Association* 272 (1994): 1592–96.

Neill, M. A. "*E. coli* O157:H7—Current Concepts and Future Prospects." *Journal of Food Safety* 10 (1989): 99–106.

Nestle, Marion. "The Spinach Fallout: Restoring Trust in California Produce." *San Jose Mercury News*, October 22, 2006.

Pappano, Laura. "Tainted Burgers Trigger New Safety Efforts." *Boston Globe*, February 17, 1993.

Pollock, G. J., D. Young, T. J. Beattie, and W. T. A. Todd. "Clinical Surveillance of Thrombotic Microangiopathies in Scotland, 2003–2005." *Epidemiology and Infection* 136 (2007): 115–21.

Porterfield, Elaine, and Adam Berliant. "Jack-in-the-Box Ignored Safety Rules." *The News Tribune* (Tacoma, Wash.), June 16, 1995.

Rangel, J. M., et al. "Epidemiology of *E. coli* O157:H7 Outbreaks in the United States, 1982–2002." *Emerging Infectious Diseases* 11 (2005): 603–9.

Raver, Anne. "Hooked on Cider." *New York Times*, October 31, 1993.

Repetto, H. A. "Epidemic Hemolytic-Uremic Syndrome in Children." *Kidney International* 52 (1997): 1708–19.

Riley, L. W., et al. "Hemorrhagic Colitis Associated with a Rare *E. coli* Serotype." *New England Journal of Medicine* 308 (1983): 681–85.

Roessingh, A. S. de Buys, et al. "Gastrointestinal Complications of Post-Diarrheal Hemolytic Uremic Syndrome." *European Journal of Pediatric Surgery* 17 (2007): 328–34.

Safdar, N., et al. "Risk of Hemolytic Uremic Syndrome After Antibiotic Treatment of *E. coli* O157:H7 Enteritis: A Meta-Analysis." *Journal of the American Medical Association* 288 (2002): 996–1001.

Salerno, A., K. Meyers, K. McGowan, and B. Kaplan. "Hemolytic Uremic Syndrome Associated with Laboratory Acquired *E. coli* O157:H7." *Journal of Pediatrics* 145 (2004): 412–14.

"Second Outbreak of Bacterial Infection Is Reported." *New York Times*, March 28, 1993, Health section.

Steele, B. T., N. Murphy, G. S. Arbus, and C. P. Rance. "An Outbreak of Hemolytic Uremic Syndrome Associated with Ingestion of Fresh Apple Juice." *Journal of Pediatrics* 101 (1982): 963–65.

Suburban Emergency Management Project. "How *Escherichia coli* O157:H7—Cause of Ongoing Contaminated Spinach Outbreak—Poisons Humans." http://www.semp.us/publications/biot_reader.php?BiotID=408 (accessed December 2007).

Sullivan, Joseph. "Single Slaughterhouse Suspected as Tainted-Meat Source." *New York Times*, July 28, 1994, Health section.

Tarr, P. I. "*E. coli* O157:H7: Clinical, Diagnostic, and Epidemiological Aspects of Human Infection." *Clinical Infectious Diseases* 20 (1995): 1–10.

Tserenpuntsag, Boldtsetseg, Hwa-Gan Chang, Perry F. Smith, and Dale L. Morse. "Hemolytic Uremic Syndrome and *E. coli* O157:H7." *Emerging Infectious Diseases* 11 (2005): 1955–57.

"US to Issue Stricter Rules on Handling Raw Meat." *New York Times*, October 31, 1993.

Varma, J. K., et al. "An Outbreak of *E. coli* O157:H7 Infection Following Exposure to a Contaminated Building." *Journal of the American Medical Association* 290 (2003): 2709–12.

Chapter 6. Two Ticks from Jersey

Adamantos, S., A. Boag, and D. Church. "Australian Tick Paralysis in a Dog Imported into the UK." *Australian Veterinary Journal* 83 (2005): 352.

Bonduell, M. "Guillain-Barré Syndrome." *Archives of Neurology* 55 (1998): 1483–85.

Daugherty, R. J., et al. "Tick Paralysis: Atypical Presentation, Unusual Location." *Pediatric Emergency Care* 21 (2005): 677–80.

Dworkin, M. S., P. C. Shoemaker, and D. E. Anderson. "Tick Paralysis: 33 Human Cases in Washington State, 1946–1996." *Clinical Infectious Diseases* 29 (1999) 1435–59.

Edlow, J. A., and D. C. McGillicuddy. "Tick Paralysis." *Infectious Diseases Clinics of North America* 22 (2008): 397–413.

Emmons, R. W., F. M. Brewster, and B. C. Nelson. "Tick-Bite in Oregon: Paralysis in California." *Western Journal of Medicine* 121 (1974): 142–43.

Felz, M. W. "The Perspicacity of Seymour Hadwen on Tick Paralysis—A Commentary." *Wilderness and Environmental Medicine* 11 (2000): 113–14.

Felz, M. W., L. A. Durden, and J. H. Oliver Jr. "Ticks Parasitizing Humans in Georgia and South Carolina." *Journal of Parasitology* 82 (1996): 505–8.

Felz, M. W., C. D. Smith, and T. R. Swift. "A Six-Year-Old Girl with Tick Paralysis." *New England Journal of Medicine* 342 (2000): 90–94.

Felz, M. W., T. R. Swift, and W. Hobbs. "Tick Paralysis in the United States: A Photographic Review." *Archives of Neurology* 57 (2000): 1071–72.

Garin, C., and A. Bujadoux. "Paralysis by Ticks, 1922." *Clinical Infectious Diseases* 16 (1993): 168–69.

"Girl's Mom Describes Tick Illness: Rare Disease Causes Paralysis in the Body." *Burlington County Times*, August 3, 2003.

Gordon, B. M., and C. C. Giza. "Tick Paralysis Presenting in an Urban Environment." *Pediatric Neurology* 30 (2004): 122–24.

Gorman, R. J., and O. C. Snead. "Tick Paralysis in Three Children: The Diversity of Neurologic Presentations." *Clinical Pediatrics (Philadelphia)* 17 (1998): 249–51.

Grattan-Smith, P. J., et al. "Clinical and Neurophysiological Features of Tick Paralysis." *Brain* 120 (1997): 1975–87.

Greenstein, P. "Tick Paralysis." *Medical Clinics of North America* 86 (2003): 441–46.

Hadwen, Seymour. "Excerpts from: On 'Tick Paralysis' in Sheep and Man Following Bites of *Dermacentor venustus.*" *Wilderness and Environmental Medicine* 11 (2000): 115–21.

Helem, Lisa. "County Girl Affected by Tick Paralysis." *Burlington County Times,* August 1, 2003.

Hester, Tom. "State Issues New Tick Warning." NJ.com (August 1, 2003).

Inokuma, H., et al., "Tick Paralysis by *Ixodes holocyclus* in a Japanese Traveler Returning from Australia." *Annals of the New York Academy of Science* 990 (2003): 357–58.

Jones, H. R. Jr. "Guillain-Barré Syndrome: Perspectives with Infants and Children." *Seminars in Pediatric Neurology* 7 (2000): 91–102.

Jones, H. R. Jr. "Guillain-Barré Syndrome in Children." *Current Opinions in Pediatrics* 7 (1995): 663–68.

Li, Z., R. P. Turner. "Pediatric Tick Paralysis: Discussion of Two Cases and Literature Review." *Pediatric Neurology* 31 (2004): 304–7.

MMWR (Morbidity and Mortality Weekly Report). "Cluster of Tick Paralysis Cases—Colorado." *Journal of the American Medical Association* 55 (2006): 933–55.

MMWR (Morbidity and Mortality Weekly Report). "Tick Paralysis—Washington, 1995: From the Centers for Disease Control and Prevention." *Journal of the American Medical Association* 19 (1996): 1470.

Morris, A. M., et al. "Acute Flaccid Paralysis in Australian Children." *Journal of Pediatric and Child Health* 39 (2003): 22–26.

Morris, H. H. 3rd. "Tick Paralysis: Electrophysiologic Measurements." *Southern Medical Journal* 70 (1977): 121–22.

Pearce, J. M. S. "Octave Landry's Ascending Paralysis and the Landry-Guillain-Barré-Strohl Syndrome." *Journal of Neurology, Neurosurgery, and Psychiatry* 62 (1997): 495–500.

PhillyBurbs.com. "Caution Urged After Two Cases of Tick Paralysis." http://www.phillyburbs.com/pb-dyn/news/104-07312003-134564.html (July 31, 2003).

Rose, I. "A Review of Tick Paralysis." *Canadian Medical Association Journal* 70 (1954): 175–76.

Rucker, Angela. "State Issues Warning over Tick Diseases." *Courier-Post* (Cherry Hill, N.J.), August 1, 2003.

Schaumburg, H. H., and S. Herskovitz. "The Weak Child—Cautionary Tale." *New England Journal of Medicine* 342 (2000): 127–29.

Vedanarayanan, V. V., O. B. Evans, and S. H. Subramony. "Tick Paralysis in Children: Electrophysiology and Possibility of Misdiagnosis." *Neurology* 59 (2002): 1088–90.

Chapter 7. An Airtight Case

Arnow, P. M., J. N. Fink, D. P. Schlueter, and J. J. Barboriak, et al. "Early Detection of Hypersensitivity Pneumonitis in Office Workers." *American Journal of Medicine* 64 (1978): 236–42.

Banaszak, E. F., et al. "Epidemiologic Studies Related to Thermophilic Fungi and

Hypersensitivity Lung Syndromes." *American Review of Respiratory Diseases* 110 (1974): 585–91.

Banaszak, E. F., W. H. Thiede, and J. N. Fink. "Hypersensitivity Pneumonitis Due to Contamination of an Air Conditioner." *New England Journal of Medicine* 283 (1970): 271–76.

Campbell, J. M. "Acute Symptoms Following Work with Hay." *British Medical Journal* 2 (1932): 1143–44.

"Case Records of the Massachusetts General Hospital—Case 47-1979." *New England Journal of Medicine* 301 (1979): 1168–74.

Fink, J. N., et al. "Hypersensitivity Pneumonitis Due to Contaminated Home Environments." *Journal of Laboratory and Clinical Medicine* 78 (1971): 853–54.

Fink, J. N., et al. "Interstitial Lung Disease Due to Contamination of Forced Air Systems." *Annals of Internal Medicine* 84 (1976): 406–13.

Hanak, V., et al. "Causes and Presenting Features in 85 Patients with Hypersensitivity Pneumonitis." *Mayo Clinic Proceedings* 82 (2007): 812–16.

Kumar, P., R. Marier, and S. H. Leech. "Hypersensitivity Pneumonitis Due to Contamination of a Car Air Conditioner." *New England Journal of Medicine* 305 (1981): 1531–32.

Kumar, P., R. Marier, and S. H. Leech. "Respiratory Allergies Related to Automobile Air Conditioners." *New England Journal of Medicine* 311 (1984): 1619–21.

Linaker, C., and J. Smedley, "Respiratory Illness in Agricultural Workers." *Occupational Medicine* 52 (2002): 451–59.

Metzger, W. J., R. Patterson, J. Fink, R. Semerdjian, and M. Roberts. "Sauna-takers Disease: Hypersensitivity Pneumonitis to Contaminated Water in a Home Sauna." *Journal of the American Medical Association* 236 (1976): 2209–11.

Pepys, J. "Clinical and Therapeutic Significance of Patterns of Allergic Reactions of the Lungs to Extrinsic Agents: The 1977 J. Burns Amberson Lecture." *American Review of Respiratory Diseases* 116 (1977): 573–88.

Rickman, Otis B., Jay H. Ryu, Mary E. Fidler, and Sanjay Kalra. "Hypersensitivity Pneumonitis Associated with *Mycobacterium avium* Complex and Hot Tub Use." *Mayo Clinic Proceedings* 77 (2002): 1233–37.

Salvaggio, J. E., and R. M. Karr. "Hypersensitivity Pneumonitis: State of the Art." *Chest* 75 (1979): 270–74.

Samet, J. M., Marian C. Marbury, and J. D. Spengler. "Health Effects and Sources of Indoor Air Pollution, Part I." *American Review of Respiratory Disease* 136 (1987): 1486–1508.

Samet, J. M., Marian C. Marbury, and J. D. Spengler. "Health Effects and Sources of Indoor Air Pollution, Part II." *American Review of Respiratory Disease* 137 (1988): 221–22.

Schatz, M., R. Patterson, and J. Fink. "Immunologic Lung Disease." *New England Journal of Medicine* 300 (1979): 1310–20.

Tye, Larry. "Study: Indoor Pollution State's Worst Health Woe." *Boston Globe*, May 17, 1989.

Chapter 8. Monday Morning Fever

"Better Offer at Lawrence." *New York Times*, March 9, 1912.

Bushnell, Larry. "Beyond Polartec: Malden Mills Re-Fashions Its Identity." *Boston Globe*, February 17, 2005.

Centers for Disease Control and Prevention (CDC). "Chronic Interstitial Lung Disease in Nylon Flocking Industry Workers—Rhode Island, 1992–1996." *Morbidity and Mortality Weekly Report (MMWR)* 46 (1997): 897–901.

Centers for Disease Control and Prevention (CDC). "Polymer-Fume Fever Associated with Cigarette Smoking and the Use of Tetrafluoroethylene—Mississippi." *Morbidity and Mortality Weekly Report (MMWR)* 36 (1987): 515–16, 521–22.

Chemical Heritage Foundation. "Roy J. Plunkett." http://www.chemheritage.org/classroom/chemach/plastics/plunkett.html (accessed November 2007).

Cullen, M. R., M. G. Cherniack, and L. Rosenstock. "Occupational Medicine (1)." *New England Journal of Medicine* 322 (1990): 594–601.

Cullen, M. R., M. G. Cherniack, and L. Rosenstock. "Occupational Medicine (2)." *New England Journal of Medicine* 322 (1990): 675–83.

Daroowalla, F., et al. "Flock Workers' Exposures and Respiratory Symptoms in Five Plants." *American Journal of Industrial Medicine* 47 (2005): 144–52.

Davidoff, F. "New Disease, Old Story." *Annals of Internal Medicine* 129 (1998): 327–28.

DuPont. "History of Teflon." www.dupont.com/teflon/newsroom/history.html (accessed November 2007).

Eschenbacker, W. L., et al. "Nylon Flock-Associated Interstitial Lung Disease." *American Journal of Respiratory and Critical Care Medicine* 159 (1998): 2003–8.

Harris, D. K. "Polymer Fume Fever." *Lancet* 2 (1951): 1008–11.

Irwin, R. S., and J. M. Madison. "The Persistently Troublesome Cough." *American Journal of Respiratory and Critical Care Medicine* 165 (2002): 1469–74.

Jewell, Mark. "Prospective Malden Mills Buyer to Switch to Polartec Name." signonSanDiego.com, http://www.signonsandiego.com/news/business/20070223-1249-maldenmills-polartec.html (accessed November 2007).

Kern, David G., et al. "Flock Worker's Lung: Broadening the Spectrum of Clinicalpathology, Narrowing the Spectrum of Suspected Etiologies." *Chest* 117 (2000): 251–59.

Kern, David G., et al. "Flock-Worker's Lung: Chronic Interstitial Lung Disease in the Nylon Flocking Industry." *Annals of Internal Medicine* 129 (1998): 261–72.

Kern, David G., R. K. Kern, and K. T. Durand. "Secrecy in Science: The Flock Worker's Lung Investigation." *Annals of Internal Medicine* 130 (1999): 616.

"Lawrence Mills Increases Wages." *New York Times*, March 1, 1912.

Levy, Barry S., and D. H. Wegman, eds. *Occupational Health*. 2nd ed. Philadelphia: Lippincott Williams and Wilkins, 1989.

Lewis, C. E., and G. R. Kerby. "An Epidemic of Polymer Fume Fever." *Journal of the American Medical Association* 191 (1965): 103–6.

Morgan, Wm. Keith C., and Anthony Seaton. *Occupational Lung Disease*. Philadelphia: Saunders, 1975.

Schuchman, Miriam. "Secrecy in Science: The Flock Worker's Lung Investigation." *Annals of Internal Medicine* 129 (1998): 341–44.

"Uncovering Occupational Illnesses." *Emergency Medicine.* February 15, 1990, 22–44.

Washko, R. M., et al. "Epidemiologic Investigation of Respiratory Morbidity at a Nylon Flock Plant." *American Journal of Industrial Medicine* 38 (2000): 628–38.

Wegman, D. H., and J. M. Peter. "Polymer Fume Fever and Cigarette Smoking." *Annals of Internal Medicine* 81 (1974): 55–57.

Williams, N., and E. K. Smith. "Polymer Fume Fever: An Elusive Diagnosis." *Journal of the American Medical Association* 219 (1972): 1587–89.

Wilson, Ralph N. "The Many Faces of the Industrial Medical Officer." *Transactions of the Society of Occupational Medicine* 19 (1969): 23–26.

Chapter 9. The Case of the Wide-Eyed Boy

Adler, A. G., G. E. McElwain, G. J. Merli, and J. H. Martin. "Systemic Effects of Eye Drops." *Archives of Internal Medicine* 142 (1982): 2293–94.

Bond, D. W., H. Vyas, and H. Venning. "Mydriasis Due to Self-Administered Inhaled Ipratropium Bromide." *European Journal of Pediatrics* 161 (2002): 178.

Bryant, B. J. "*Pasteurella multocida* Bacteremia in Asymptomatic Pheresis Donors: A Tale of Two Cats." *Transfusion* 47 (2007): 1984–89.

Centers for Disease Control and Prevention (CDC). "Suspected Moonflower Intoxication—Ohio, 2002." *Morbidity and Mortality Weekly Report (MMWR)* 52 (2003): 788–91.

"Death from Nightshade Berries." *Lancet (Medical Jurisprudence section)* 48 (1846): 241.

Dryden, John, and Arthur H. Clough. "Plutarch on Antony and Cleopatra, the Last of the Ptolemies." Excerpted from Plutarch, "Antony," in *The Lives of Noble Grecians and Romans*, vol. 3 (Boston: Little, Brown, 1902). http://www.shsu.edu/~his_ncp/AntCleo.html (accessed December 2007).

Firestone, D., and C. Sloane. "Not Your Everyday Anisocoria: Angel's Trumpet Ocular Toxicity." *Journal of Emergency Medicine* 33 (2007): 21–24.

Grieve, M. "Nightshade, Deadly." Botanical.com, http://www.botanical.com/botanical/mgmh/n/nighdeo5.html (accessed November 2007).

Havelius, U., and P. Asman. "Accidental Mydriasis from Exposure to Angel's Trumpet (*Datura suaveolens*)." *Acta Ophthalmology Scandanavia* 80 (2002): 332–35.

Kulig, K., and B. H. Rumak. "Anticholinergic Poisoning." In *Winchester and Haddad's Clinical Management of Poisoning and Drug Overdose*, ed. Michael W. Shannon, Stephen W. Borron, and Michael J. Burns. Philadelphia: Saunders, 1983.

Lee, M. R. "The Solanaceae: Foods and Poisons." *Journal of the Royal College of Physicians Edinburgh* 36 (2006): 162–69.

Lee, M. R. "The Solanaceae II: The Mandrake (*Mandragora officinarum*); In League with the Devil." *Journal of the Royal College of Physicians Edinburgh* 36 (2006): 278–85.

Lee, M. R. "Solanaceae III: Henbane, Hags, and Hawley Harvey Crippen." *Journal of the Royal College of Physicians Edinburgh* 36 (2006): 366–73.

Lee, M. R. "Solanaceae IV: *Atropa belladonna*, Deadly Nightshade." *Journal of the Royal College of Physicians Edinburgh* 37 (2007): 77–84.

Meng, K., and D. K. Graetz. "Moonflower-Induced Anisocoria." *Annals of Emergency Medicine* 44 (2004): 665–66.

Proudfoot, A. "Early Toxicology of Physostigmine: A Tale of Beans, Great Men, and Egos." *Toxicology Reviews* 25 (2000): 98–138.

Raman, S. V., and J. Jacob. "Mydriasis Due to *Datura inoxia*." *Emergency Medicine Journal* 22 (2005): 310–11.

Roberts, J. R. "Pseudo Cerebral Herniation Syndrome Due to Phenylephrine Nasal Spray." *New England Journal of Medicine* 320 (1989): 1757.

Rosen, N. B. "Accidental Mydriasis from Scopolamine Patches." *Journal of the American Optometric Association* 57 (1986): 541–42.

Taylor, Norman. *Plant Drugs that Changed the World*. London: Allen and Unwin, 1966.

Thiele, E. A., and J. J. Riviello. "Scopolamine Patch-Induced Unilateral Mydriasis." *Pediatrics* 93 (1985): 525.

Toscano, A., C. Pancaro, and V. A. Peduto. "Scopolamine Prevents Dreams During General Anesthesia." *Anesthesiology* 106 (2007): 952–55.

Voltz, R., R. Hohlfeld, M. Liebler, and H. Hertel. "Gardener's Mydriasis." *Lancet* 339 (1992): 752.

Weir, R., D. Whitehead, F. Zaidi, and B. Greaves. "Pupil Blown by a Puffer." *Lancet* 364 (2004): 415.

Chapter 10. A Study in Scarlet

Attaran, R. R., and F. Probst. "Histamine Fish Poisoning: A Common but Frequently Misdiagnosed Condition." *Emergency Medical Journal* 19 (2002): 474–75.

Bartholomew, B. A., P. R. Berry, J. C. Rodhouse, and R. J. Gilbert. "Scombrotoxic Fish Poisoning in Britain: Features of over 250 Suspected Incidents from 1976–1986." *Epidemiology and Infection* 99 (1987): 775–82.

Borade, P., C. Ballary, and D. Lee. "A Fishy Cause of Sudden Near Fatal Hypotension." *Resuscitation* 72 (2007): 158–60.

Centers for Disease Control and Prevention (CDC). "Scombroid Fish Poisoning Associated with Tuna Steaks." *Morbidity and Mortality Weekly Report (MMWR)* 56 (2007): 817–19.

Centers for Disease Control and Prevention (CDC). "Scombroid Fish Poisoning— Illinois and Michigan." *Morbidity and Mortality Weekly Report (MMWR)* 29 (1980): 167–68.

Centers for Disease Control and Prevention (CDC). "Scombroid Fish Poisoning— Illinois and South Carolina." *Morbidity and Mortality Weekly Report (MMWR)* 38 (1989): 140–42, 147.

Centers for Disease Control and Prevention (CDC). "Scombroid Fish Poisoning— New Mexico." *Morbidity and Mortality Weekly Report (MMWR)* 37 (1989): 451.

Centers for Disease Control and Prevention (CDC). "Scombroid Poisoning—New Jersey." *Morbidity and Mortality Weekly Report (MMWR)* 29 (1980): 106–7.

Etkind, P., M. E. Wilson, K. Gallagher, and J. Cournoyer. "Bluefish-Associated Scombroid Poisoning, an Example of the Expanding Spectrum of Food Poisoning from Seafood." *Journal of the American Medical Association* 258 (1987): 3409–10.

Feldman, K. A., et al. "A Large Outbreak of Scombroid Fish Poisoning Associated with Eating Escolar Fish (*Lepidocybium flavobrunneum*)." *Epidemiology of Infections* 133 (2004): 29–33.

Food-Service Establishment Inspection Reports. Prepared by John K. Seiferth, of the Department of Health and Human Services of the State of New Hampshire, prepared June 5, 1985, October 7, 1985, and July 24, 1986.

Gellert, G. A., et al. "Scombroid Fish Poisoning: Underreporting and Prevention Among Noncommercial Recreational Fishers." *Western Journal of Medicine* 157 (1992): 645–47.

Grinda, Jean-Michel, et al. "Biventricular Assist Device for Scombroid Poisoning with Refractory Myocardial Dysfunction: A Bridge to Recovery." *Critical Care Medicine* 32 (2004): 1957–59.

McInerney, J., et al. "Scombroid Poisoning." *Annals of Emergency Medicine* 28 (1996): 235–38.

Saltman, Avi. "Fading Foliage." *New York Times*, October 16, 2005, New York and Region section.

Scombroid Poisoning. Public Health Bulletin (Britain), prepared May 2001.

Thoreau, Henry David. "Autumnal Tints." *Atlantic Monthly*, October 1862.

Wallace, B. J., et al. "Seafood-Associated Disease Outbreaks in New York, 1980–1994—Implications for Control." *American Journal of Preventative Medicine* 17 (1999): 48–54.

Weinheimer, Monica. "Family Scombridae: Albacores, Bonitos, Mackerels, and Tunas." *University of Michigan Museum of Zoology, Animal Diversity Web*, http://animaldiversity.ummz.umich.edu/site/accounts/information/Scombroidae (accessed November 2007).

Chapter 11. The Case of the Overly Hot Honeymoon

Ahmed, A. H., and N. H. Ahmed. "History of Disorders of Thyroid Function." *Eastern Mediterranean Health Journal* 11 (2005): 1–12.

American Thyroid Association. www.thyroid.org.

Becker, W. F. "Pioneers in Thyroid Surgery." *Annals of Surgery* 185 (1977): 493–504.

Carpenter, Kenneth J. "David Marine and the Problem of Goiter." *Journal of Nutrition* 135 (2005): 675–80.

DuBose, J. "Honest and Sensible Surgeons: The History of Thyroid Surgery." *Current Surgery* 61 (2004): 213–19.

Giddings, A. E. "The History of Thyroidectomy." *Journal of the Royal Society of Medicine* 91 (1998): 3–6.

Greer, M. A. "Daruma Eyes: The Sixth-Century Founder of Zen Buddhism and Kung Fu Had the Earliest Recorded Graves' Ophthalmopathy." *Thyroid* 12 (2002): 389–91.

Handcock, J. Duffy. "The Irish School of Medicine." Paper presented to the Innominate Society at the University of Louisville School of Medicine, 1928. http://www.innominatesociety.com/Articles/The%20Irish%20School%20of %20Medicine.htm (accessed in November 2007).

Harwick, R. D. "Our Legacy of Thyroid Surgery." *American Journal of Surgery* 156 (1988): 230–34.

Jay, V. "A Portrait in History: Dr. Robert Graves." *Archives of Pathology and Laboratory Medicine* 123 (1999): 283–84.

MacCallum, W. G. "William Stewart Halsted." *National Academy of Sciences Biographical Memoirs* 17 (1935): 151–70.

McKenna, T. J. "Graves' Disease." *Lancet* 357 (2001): 1793–96.

Nelson, C. W. "The Surgical Career of the Mayo Brothers." *Mayo Clinic Proceedings* 73 (1998): 716.

Perrier, N. D., and M. S. Boger. "Medicine's Greatest Gifts to Surgery." *World Journal of Surgery* 28 (2004): 1057–59.

Perzik, S. L. "The Place of Total Thyroidectomy in the Management of 909 Patients with Thyroid Disease." *American Journal of Surgery* 132 (1976): 480–83.

Ritchie, W. P., et al., "Workloads and Practice Patterns of General Surgeons in the United States: 1995–1997." *Annals of Surgery* 230 (1999): 533–43.

Rosen, Irving B. "A Historical Note on Thyroid Disease and Its Surgical Treatment." *Canadian Thyroid Cancer Support Group (Thry'vors) Inc.*, April 2006.

Sawin, Clark T. "What Causes Tetany After Removal of the Parathyroid Glands? MacCallum, Voegtlin, and Calcium." *The Endocrinologist* 13 (2003): 1–3.

Stellhorn, C. E. "Robert James Graves." *American Journal of Surgery* (April 1935): 183–89.

Tapscott, W. J. "A Brief History of Thyroid Surgery." *Current Surgery* 58 (2001): 464–67.

Vellar, I. D. "Thomas Peel Dunhill, the Forgotten Man of Thyroid Surgery." *Medical History* 18 (1974): 22–50.

Weetman, A. P. "Graves' Disease." *Hormone Research* 59 (suppl) (2003): 114–18.

Weitzman, S. A., et al. "Antineutrophil Auto-Antibodies in Graves' Disease." *Journal of Clinical Investigation* 75 (1984): 119–23.

Whitehead, Richard W. "Robert James Graves—Physician, Educator, and Scientist." *Circulation* 39 (1969): 719–21.

Who Named It. "Robert James Graves." http://www.whonamedit.com/doctor.cfm/ 695.html (accessed December 2007).

Chapter 12. Feeling His Oats

Altman, Lawrence. "Dr. Denis Burkitt Is Dead at 82; Thesis Changed Diets of Millions." *New York Times*, April 16, 1993, Obituary.

Anderson, J. W., and J. Tietyen-Clark. "Dietary Fiber: Hyperlipidemia, Hypertension, and Coronary Heart Disease." *American Journal of Gastroenterology* 81 (1986): 907–15.

Andrus, C. H., and J. L. Ponsky. "Bezoars: Classification, Pathophysiology, and Treatment." *American Journal of Gastroenterology* 83 (1988): 476–78.

Burkitt, D. P., et al. "Dietary Fiber and Disease." *Journal of the American Medical Association* 229 (1974): 1068–74.

Burstein, I., R. Steinberg, and M. Zer. "Small Bowel Obstruction and Covered Perforation in Childhood Caused by Bizarre Bezoars and Foreign Bodies." *Israel Medical Association Journal* 2 (2000): 129–31.

Chintamani, R. D., et al. "Cotton Bezoar—A Rare Cause of Intestinal Obstruction: Case Report." *BMC Surgery* 3 (2003): 5.

Cooper, S. G., and E. J. Tracey. "Small Bowel Obstruction Due to Oat Bran Bezoar." *New England Journal of Medicine* 320 (1989): 1148–49.

Cnn.com/health. "Doctors Untangle the Strange Case of the Giant Hairball." November 22, 2007. http://edition.cnn.com/2007/HEALTH/11/21/hairball.case/index.html (accessed December 2007).

"Fiber in the Diet." *Time Magazine*, editorial, September 2, 1974.

GG Bran Crispbread. "Lower Cholesterol Dietary Fiber." http://www.brancrisp bread.com/articles/lower_cholesterol_dietary_fiber.html.

Goldstein, S. S., J. H. Lewis, and R. Rothstein. "Intestinal Obstruction Due to Bezoars." *American Journal of Gastroenterology* 79 (1984): 313–18.

Hillips, M. R., S. Zaheer, and G. T. Drugas. "Gastric Trichobezoar: Case Report and Literature Review." *Mayo Clinic Proceedings* 73 (1996): 653–55.

Ho, T. W., and D. C. Koh, "Small Bowel Obstruction Secondary to Bezoar Obstruction: A Diagnostic Dilemma." *World Journal of Surgery* 31 (2007): 1072–78.

Holland, B. K. "Treatments for Bubonic Plague: Treatments from 17th-Century British Epidemics." *Journal of the Royal Society of Medicine* 93 (2000): 322–24.

Kishan, A. S. N., et al. "Bezoars." *British History Journal* (October 2000). http://www.bhj.org/journal/2001_4304_oct/org_507.htm.

Kövi, R., E. Kis, and I. K. Várkonyi. "Difficulties in the Diagnosis of Bezoars." *Yearbook of Pediatric Radiology: Current Problems in Pediatric Radiology*, ed. Bela Lombay. 1999.

Kowalski, Robert E. *The Eight-Week Cholesterol Cure: How to Lower Your Blood Cholesterol by Up to 40 Percent Without Drugs or Deprivation.* New York: Harper and Row, 1987.

Liu, Simin. "Whole-Grain Foods, Dietary Fiber, and Type 2 Diabetes: Searching for a Kernel of Truth." *American Journal of Clinical Nutrition* 77 (2003): 527–29.

Malcom, Corey. "Bezoar Stones." *The Navigator: Newsletter of the Mel Fisher Maritime Heritage Society* 13(6) (June 1998).

Marlett, J. A., M. I. McBurney, and J. L. Slavin. "Position of the American Dietetic Association: Health Implications of Dietary Fiber." *Journal of the American Dietetic Association* 102 (2002): 993–1000.

Milov, David E., Joel M. Andres, Nora A. Erhart, and David J. Bailey. "Chewing Gum Bezoars of the Gastrointestinal Tract." *Pediatrics* 102 (1998): e22–24.

Moor, Thomas. "The Cholesterol Myth." *The Atlantic*, September 1989, 264.

MUSC Digestive Disease Center. http://www.ddc.musc.edu/ddc_pro/pro_development/case_studies/case040.htm (accessed December 2007).

Pitiakoudis, Michail, Alexandra Tsaroucha, Konstantinos Mimidis, and Theodoros

Constantinidis. "Esophageal and Small Bowel Obstruction by Occupational Bezoar." *BMC Gastroenterology* 3 (2003): 13–17.

Story, Jon A., and David Kritchevky. "Denis Parsons Burkitt (1911–1993)." *Journal of Nutrition* 124 (1994): 1551–54.

Vitellas, Kenneth M., William F. Bennett, Kuldeep Vaswani, and Sangeeta Guttikonda. "Gastrointestinal Case of the Day." *American Journal of Radiology* 175 (2000): 872–79.

Yau, Kwok Kay, et al. "Laparoscopic Approach Compared with Conventional Open Approach to Bezoar-Induced Small Bowel Obstruction." *Archives of Surgery* 140 (2005): 972–75.

Chapter 13. The Case of the Unhealthy Health Food

Altaee, M. Y., and M. H. Mahmood. "An Outbreak of Veno-Occlusive Disease of the Liver in Northern Iraq." *Eastern Mediterranean Health Journal* 4 (1998): 142–48.

Aydinili, M., and Y. Bayraktar. "Budd-Chiari Syndrome: Etiology, Pathogenesis, and Diagnosis." *World Journal of Gastroenterology* 13 (2007): 2693–96.

Bach, N., S. N. Thung, and F. Schaffner. "Comfrey Herb Tea-Induced Hepatic Veno-Occlusive Disease." *American Journal of Medicine* 87 (1989): 97–99.

Bergner, Paul. "Symphytum: Comfrey, Coltsfoot, and Pyrrolizidine Alkaloids." *Medical Herbalism: Materia Medica and Pharmacy* 2001, http://medherb.com/Materia_Medica/Symphytum_-_Comfrey,_Coltsfoot,_and_Pyrrolizidine_Alkaloids.htm (accessed November 2007).

Bras, G. "Some Investigations into Liver Disease in the West Indies: Historic Overview." *West Indian Medical Journal* 23 (1974): 160–64.

Bras, G., et al. "Veno-Occlusive Disease of Liver with Nonportal Type of Cirrhosis, Occurring in Jamaica." *Archives of Pathology* 57 (1954): 285–300.

Bras, G., D. M. Berry, and P. Gyorgy. "Plants as Aetiological Factor in Veno-Occlusive Disease of the Liver." *Lancet* 272 (1957): 960–62.

Bras, G., S. E. H. Brooks, and D. C. Watler. "Cirrhosis of the Liver in Jamaica." *Journal of Pathology and Bacteriology* 82 (1961): 503–12.

Bras, G., D. B. Jelliffe, and K. L. Stuart. "Veno-Occlusive Disease of the Liver." *Pediatrics* 14 (1954): 334–39.

Brooks, S. E., et al. "Acute Veno-Occlusive Disease of the Liver: Fine Structure in Jamaican Children." *Archives of Pathology* 89 (1970): 507–20.

Chitturi, S., and G. C. Farrell. "Herbal Hepatotoxicity: An Expanding but Poorly Defined Problem." *Journal of Gastroenterology and Hepatology* 15 (2000): 1093–99.

Dai, N. "Gynura Root Induces Hepatic Veno-Occlusive Disease: A Case Report and Review of the Literature." *World Journal of Gastroenterology* 14 (2007): 1628–31.

Dickinson, J. O., M. P. Cooke, R. R. King, and P. A. Mohamed. "Milk Transfer of Pyrrolizidine Alkaloids in Cattle." *Journal of the American Veterinary Medical Association* 169 (1976): 1192–96.

Fogden, E., and J. Neuberger. "Alternative Medicines and the Liver." *Liver International* 23 (2003): 213–20.

Furbee, R. B. "Hepatotoxicity Associated with Herbal Products." *Clinical and Laboratory Medicine* 1 (2006): 227–41.

Goleman, Daniel. "Shaman's Plant Lore May Die with Forests." *New York Times*, June 11, 1991, Health section.

Guan, Yong-Song. "A Case Report of Hepatic Veno-Occlusive Disease After Ingesting Dainties." *World Journal of Gastroenterology* 12 (2006): 6734–35.

Jelliffe, D. B., G. Bras, and K. L. Stuart. "The Clinical Picture of Veno-Occlusive Disease of the Liver in Jamaican Children." *Annals of Tropical Medicine and Parasitology* 48 (1954): 386–96.

Jelliffe, Derrick B., Gerrit Bras, and Kanai L. Mukherjee. "Veno-Occlusive Disease of the Liver and Indian Childhood Cirrhosis." *Archives of Diseases of Childhood* 32 (1957): 369–85.

Koff, R. S. "Herbal Hepatotoxicity: Revisiting a Dangerous Alternative." *Journal of the American Medical Association* 273 (1995): 502.

Kumana, C. R., et al. "Hepatic Veno-Occlusive Disease Due to Toxic Alkaloid Herbal Tea." *Lancet* 2 (1983): 1360–61.

Kumana, C. R., et al. "Herbal Tea Induced Hepatic Veno-Occlusive Disease: Quantification of Toxic Alkaloid Exposure in Adults." *Gut* 26 (1985): 101–14.

Larrey, D. "Hepatotoxicity of Herbal Remedies." *Journal of Hepatology* 26 Supplement 1 (1997): 47–51.

Lewis, W. H. "Reporting Adverse Reactions to Herbal Ingestants." *Journal of the American Medical Association* 240 (1978): 109–10.

Lewis, W. H., and P. R. Smith. "Poke Root Herbal Tea Poisoning." *Journal of the American Medical Association* 242 (1979): 2759–60.

McDermott, W. V., and P. M. Ridker. "The Budd-Chiari Syndrome and Hepatic Veno-Occlusive Disease Recognition and Treatment." *Archives of Surgery* 125 (1990): 525–27.

McDermott, W. V., M. D. Stone, A. Bothe Jr., and C. Trey. "Budd-Chiari Syndrome: Historical and Clinical Review with an Analysis of Surgical Corrective Procedures." *American Journal of Surgery* 147 (1984): 463–67.

McGee, J., R. S. Patrick, C. B. Wood, and L. H. Blumgart. "A Case of Veno-Occlusive Disease of the Liver in Britain Associated with Herbal Tea Consumption." *Journal of Clinical Pathology* 29 (1976): 788–94.

MacGregor, F. B., et al. "Hepatotoxicity of Herbal Remedies." *British Medical Journal* 299 (1989): 1156–57.

Mattocks, A. R. "Toxicity of Pyrrolizidine Alkaloids." *Nature* 217 (1968): 723–28.

Mattocks, A. R. "Toxic Pyrrolizidine Alkaloids in Comfrey." *Lancet* 2 (1980): 1136–37.

Mattocks, A. R., and R. Jukes. "Improved Field Tests for Toxic Pyrrolizidine Alkaloids." *Journal of Natural Products* 50 (1987): 161–66.

Mattocks, A. R., and I. N. White. "Pyrrolic Metabolites from Non-Toxic Pyrrolizidine Alkaloids." *Natural New Biology* 231 (1971): 114–15.

Miller, L. G. "Herbal Medicinals." *Archives of Internal Medicine* 158 (1998): 2200–2211.

Mitchell, M. C., et al. "Budd-Chiari Syndrome: Etiology, Diagnosis, and Management." *Medicine (Baltimore)* 61 (1982): 199–218.

Mohabbat, O., et al. "An Outbreak of Hepatic Veno-Occlusive Disease in North-Western Afghanistan." *Lancet* 2 (1976): 269–71.

Okuda, K., M. Kage, and S. Shrestha. "Proposal of a New Nomenclature for Budd-Chiari Syndrome: Hepatic Vein Thrombosis Versus Thrombosis of the Inferior Vena Cava at Its Hepatic Portion." *Hepatology* 28 (1998): 1191–98.

Pak, Eddy, Karl Esrason, and Victor H. Wu. "Hepatotoxicity of Herbal Remedies: An Emerging Dilemma." *Progress in Transplantation* 14 (2004): 91–96.

Parker, R. G. "Occlusion of the Hepatic Veins in Man." *Medicine (Baltimore)* 38 (1959): 369–402.

Reuben, A. "Illustrious, Industrious, and Perhaps Notorious." *Hepatology* 38 (2003): 1064–69.

Reuben, A. "My Cup Runneth Over." *Hepatology* 38 (2004): 503–7.

Ridker, P. M., et al. "Hepatic Venocclusive Disease Associated with the Consumption of Pyrrolizidine-Containing Dietary Supplements." *Gastroenterology* 88 (1985): 1050–54.

Ridker, P. M., et al. "Hepatic Veno-Occlusive Disease and Herbal Teas." *Journal of Pediatrics* 115 (1989): 167.

Ridker, P. M., and W. V. McDermott. "Comfrey Herb Tea and Hepatic Veno-Occlusive Disease." *Lancet* 1 (1989): 657–58.

Ridker, P. M., and W. V. McDermott. "Hepatotoxicity Due to Comfrey Herb Tea." *American Journal of Medicine* 87 (1989): 701.

Roitman, J. N. "Comfrey and Liver Damage." *Lancet* 1 (1981): 944.

Rollins, B. J., et al. "Hepatic Veno-Occlusive Disease." *American Journal of Medicine* 2 (1986): 297–306.

Roulet, M., R. Laurini, L. Rivier, and L. A. Calame. "Hepatic Veno-Occlusive Disease in Newborn Infant of a Woman Drinking Herbal Tea." *Journal of Pediatrics* 112 (1988): 433–36.

Routledge, P. A., and T. L. Spriggs. "Atropine as Possible Contaminant of Comfrey Tea." *Lancet* 1 (1989): 963–64.

Schoental, R., and A. R. Mattocks. "Hepatotoxic Activity of Semi-Synthetic Analogues of Pyrrolizidine Alkaloids." *Nature* 185 (1960): 842–43.

Schoepfer, A. M., et al. "Herbal Does Not Mean Innocuous: Ten Cases of Severe Hepatotoxicity Associated with Dietary Supplements from Herbalife Products." *Journal of Hepatology* 4 (2007): 521–26.

Seeff, L. B. "Herbal Hepatotoxicity." *Clinical Liver Disease* 11 (2007): 577–96.

Selzer, G., and R. G. Parker. "Senecio Poisoning Exhibiting as Chiari's Syndrome: A Report on Twelve Cases." *American Journal of Pathology* 27 (1951): 885–907.

Stedman, Catherine. "Herbal Hepatotoxicity." *Seminars in Liver Disease* 2 (2002): 195–206.

Stickel, F., and D. Schuppan. "Herbal Hepatotoxicity." *Journal of Hepatology* 5 (2005): 901–10.

Stickel, F., and H. K. Seitz. "The Efficacy and Safety of Comfrey." *Public Health Nutrition* 3 (2000): 501–8.

Stillman, A. S., et al. "Hepatic Veno-Occlusive Disease Due to Pyrrolizidine (Senecio) Poisoning in Arizona." *Gastroenterology* 12 (1977): 349–52.

Stuart, K. L., and G. Bras. "Veno-Occlusive Disease of the Liver." *Quarterly Journal of Medicine* 26 (1957): 291–315.

Subiza, J., et al. "Anaphylactic Reaction After the Ingestion of Chamomile Tea: A Study of Cross-Reactivity with Other Composite Pollens." *Journal of Allergy and Clinical Immunology* 84 (1989): 353–58.

Tandon, H. D., B. N. Tandon, and A. R. Mattocks. "An Epidemic of Veno-Occlusive Disease of the Liver in Afghanistan: Pathologic Features." *American Journal of Gastroenterology* 70 (1978): 607–13.

University of Maryland Medical Center. "Comfrey." http://www.umm.edu/altmed/articles/comfrey-000234.htm (accessed November 2007).

Weston, C. F., B. T. Cooper, J. D. Davies, and D. F. Levine. "Veno-Occlusive Disease of the Liver Secondary to Ingestion of Comfrey." *British Medical Journal (Clinical Resource Ed)* 295 (1987): 183.

Willett, Kristine L., Robert A. Roth, and Larry Walker. "Workshop Overview: Hepatotoxicity Assessment for Botanical Dietary Supplements." *Toxicological Sciences* 79 (2004): 4–9.

Zuckerman, M., V. Steenkamp, and J. Stewart. "Hepatic Veno-Occlusive Disease as a Result of a Traditional Remedy: Confirmation of Toxic Pyrrolizidine Alkaloids as the Cause, Using an In-Vitro Technique." *Journal of Clinical Pathology* 55 (2002): 676–79.

Chapter 14. Little Luisa's Blinding Headache

Baker, R. S., R. J. Baumann, and J. R. Buncic. "Idiopathic Intracranial Hypertension in Pediatric Patients." *Pediatric Neurology* 5 (1989): 5–11.

Ball, A. K., and C. E. Clarke. "Idiopathic Intracranial Hypertension." *Lancet Neurology* 5 (2006): 433–42.

Binder, D. K., et al. "Idiopathic Intracranial Hypertension." *Neurosurgery* 54 (2004): 538–52.

Carrington-Smith, Denise. "Mawson and Mertz: A Re-Evaluation of Their Ill-Fated Mapping Journey During the 1911–1914 Australasian Antarctic Exploration." *Medical Journal of Australia* 183 (2005): 638–41.

Donohue, Sean P. "Recurrence of Idiopathic Intracranial Hypertension After Weight Loss: The Carrot Craver." *American Journal of Ophthalmology* 116 (2000) 850–51.

Galvin, Jennifer A., and Gregory P. Van Staver. "Clinical Characterization of Idiopathic Intracranial Hypertension at the Detroit Medical Center." *Journal of the Neurological Sciences* 223 (2004): 157–60.

Hathcock, J. N., et al. "Evaluation of Vitamin A Toxicity" *American Journal of Clinical Nutrition* 52 (1990): 183–203.

Jacobson, D. M., et al. "Serum Vitamin A Concentration Is Elevated in Idiopathic Intracranial Hypertension." *Neurology* 53 (1999): 1114–20.

Johnston, I. "The Historical Development of the Pseudotumor Concept." *Neurosurgical Focus* 11 (2001): 1–9.

Johnston, Ian, Brian Owler, and John Pickard. *The Pseudotumor Cerebri Syndrome.* Cambridge: Cambridge University Press, 2007. Chapters 1–4.

Lam, H. S., et al. "Risk of Vitamin A Toxicity from Candy-Like Chewable Vitamin Supplements for Children." *Pediatrics* 118 (2006): 820–24.

Lim, M. "Visual Failure Without Headache in Idiopathic Intracranial Hypertension." *Archives of the Diseases of Childhood* 90 (2005): 206–10.

Penniston, K. L., and S. A. Tanumihardjo. "The Acute and Chronic Toxic Effects of Vitamin A." *American Journal of Clinical Nutrition* 83 (1991): 191–201.

Rangwala, L. M., and G. G. Liu. "Pediatric Idiopathic Intracranial Hypertension." *Survey of Ophthalmology* 52(6) (2007): 596–617.

T. E. C. Jr. "Dr. Arthur Wentworth and the First Lumbar Puncture at the Boston Children's Hospital in 1895." *Pediatrics* 62 (1978): 401.

Warman, R. "Management of Pseudotumor Cerebri in Children." *International Pediatrics* 15 (2000): 147–50.

Who Named It. "Heinrich Irenaeus Quincke." http://www.whonamedit.com/doctor .cfm/504.html (accessed December 2007).

Chapter 15. Too Much of a Good Thing

Barrueto, F. "Acute Vitamin D Intoxication in a Child." *Pediatrics* 116 (2005): e453–56.

Bertrand, Paul P., and Rebecca L. Bertrand. "Teaching Basic Gastrointestinal Physiology Using Classic Papers by WB Cannon." *Advances in Physiology Education* 31 (2007): 136–39.

Carpenter, K. J., and L. Zhao. "Forgotten Mysteries in the Early History of Vitamin D." *Journal of Nutrition* 129 (1999): 923–27.

Conlan, Roberta, and Elizabeth Sherman. "Unraveling the Enigma of Vitamin D." *National Academy of Sciences,* http://www.beyonddiscovery.org/content/view.txt .asp?a=414 (accessed November 2007).

DeLuca, H. F. "The Vitamin D Story: A Collaborative Effort of Basic Science and Clinical Medicine." *Federation of American Societies for Experimental Biology* 2 (1988): 224–36.

Dolev, Eran. "A Gland in Search of Function: The Role of the Parathyroid Glands and the Explanation of Tetany—1903–1926." *Journal of the History of Medicine and Allied Sciences* 42 (1987): 186–98.

Gosselin, Peter. "Sharon Case Shows Gap in Milk Safety." *Boston Globe,* July 21, 1991.

Holick, Michael R. "Vitamin D Deficiency." *New England Journal of Medicine* 357 (2007): 266–81.

Jacobus, C. H., et al. "Hypervitaminosis D Associated with Drinking Milk." *New England Journal of Medicine* 326 (192): 1173–77.

Jones, Richard. "19 of 1,630 Tested After Dairy Mistake." *Boston Globe,* July 18, 1991.

Jung, Helen. "Customers of Sharon Dairy Urged to Take Test for Calcium Levels." *Boston Globe,* July 4, 1991.

Jung, Helen. "Ex-Clients Hit Dairy on Milk Taint." *Boston Globe,* July 17, 1991.

Lett, Susan M. Public Health Alerts from the Commonwealth of Massachusetts Department of Public Health of July 12 and July 15, 1991.

Mitchell, H. H., T. S. Hamilton, F. R. Steggerda, and H. W. Bean. "The Chemical Composition of the Adult Human Body and Its Bearing on the Biochemistry of Growth." *Journal of Biological Chemistry* (1945): 625–37.

"New Publications: What Is Nature Doing? *Evolution and Disease*, by J. Bland-Sutton." Book Review, *New York Times*, August 25, 1890.

O'Riordan, Jeffrey L. H. "Rickets in the 17th Century." *Journal of Bone and Mineral Metabolism* 21 (2006): 1506–10.

Rajakumar, K. "Vitamin D, Cod-Liver Oil, Sunlight, and Rickets: A Historical Perspective." *Pediatrics* 112 (2003): e132–35.

Rajakumar, K., and S. B. Thomas. "Re-Emerging Nutritional Rickets: A Historical Perspective." *Archives of Pediatrics* 159 (2005): 335–41.

Seer's Training Web Site. "Body Functions." http://training.seer.cancer.gov/module _anatomy/unit1_2_body_functions.html (accessed December 2007).

Staunton, Vanee. "Family Sues Dairy." *Boston Globe*, July 13, 1991.

Stein, Rob. "Vitamin D Deficiency Called Major Health Risk." *Washington Post*, May 21, 2004.

Szurskewski, J. H. "A 100 Year Perspective on Gastrointestinal Motility." *American Journal of Physiology* 274 (1998): 447–53.

Thomson, R. B., and J. K. Johnson. "Another Family with Acute Vitamin D Intoxication: Another Cause of Familial Hypercalcemia." *Postgraduate Medical Education* 62 (1986): 1025–28.

Toni, R. "Ancient Views on the Hypothalamic-Pituitary-Thyroid Axis: A Historical and Epistemological Perspective." *Pituitary* 3 (2000): 83–98.

Vieth, R. "Vitamin D Supplementation, 25-hydroxyvitamin D Concentrations and Safety." *American Journal of Clinical Nutrition* 69 (1999): 842–56.

Vitamin D Home Page, University of California, Riverside. "History of Vitamin D." http://vitamind.ucr.edu/history.html (accessed November 2007).

Who Named It? "Claude Bernard." www.whonamedit.com (accessed November 2007).

Who Named It? "Walter Bradford Cannon." www.whonamedit.com (accessed November 2007).

Wilton, P. "Cod-Liver Oil, Vitamin D, and the Fight Against Rickets." *Canadian Medical Association Journal* 152 (1995): 1516–17.

Wolf, George. "The Discovery of Vitamin D: The Contribution of Adolf Windaus." *Journal of Nutrition* 134 (2004): 1299–1302.

Index

Bedford Village, New York, 10
Bell's palsy, 78
Belmont, Massachusetts, 197
Bernard, Claude, 131, 133, 143, 198–99
Besser, Richard, 66–67, 69–70
bezoars, 161–64, 168
Biafran war, 97
Bland-Sutton, James, 203
blood urea nitrogen (BUN), 60
blown cans, 8
bluefish, 133, 135–39
Bolshevik Revolution, 191
Bon Vivant, 10
Boston City Hospital, 20
Boston Globe, 208
Boston University School of Medicine, 201
botox, 11
Bottone, Edward J., 46–49, 53–57
botulism, 5–17, 43
    infant, 11
    types A, B, and C, 9, 15–16
    wound, 11
botulus, 5
bowel obstruction, 159–60
Bowen, Walter, 29
brass fever, 109
brass founders' ague, 109
breast cancer, 46
British Columbia Department of Agriculture, 84
British Journal of Homeopathy, 161
British Medical Journal, 92
Brompton Hospital, 95
bronchial tube constriction, 142
Brown University School of Medicine, 113
bruits, 119
Bureau of Labor Statistics, 104
Burkitt, Denis, 165–66
BZ (chemical agent), 125

cadaverine, 136, 139
calcipotriene, 206
Cambridge, Massachusetts, 116, 134, 166
Campbell, J. Munro, 92, 93
campylobacter, 36, 60
cancer, 20, 46, 50, 88–89, 91, 127, 145, 163, 165–66, 172–75, 193, 200–201
canned corned beef, 22
Cannon, Walter B., 199
Cape Girardeau, Missouri, 34–36
cardiac arrest, 40, 116
carrier (carrier state), 22–23, 27–28, 30–31, 33
carrots, 9, 195
Castleberry, 10
catheter, 62, 65, 68, 85, 121, 174
Catskills, 3, 18, 31–32
cellulitis, 34, 43
Centers for Disease Control and Prevention (CDC), 12–15, 25, 35, 38, 51–52, 62, 77, 81, 87, 97, 137
Central America, 21, 32
cerebrospinal fluid, 81, 119, 191–92
Chandelor v. Lopus, 162
chemotherapy, 50, 127
Chick, Harriet, 203
chicken pox, 47–49
Children's Hospital Boston, 65–66, 127, 185, 190
Children's Hospital of Philadelphia (CHOP), 75
Chilean Andes, 122
Chinese okra. *See* loofah
cholera, 35, 37–38, 60
cholesterol, 158, 164–67
cholestyramine, 164
Christie, A. Barnett, 5–6, 9
ciguatera poisoning, 43
Civil War, 20
Cleopatra, 122, 124

infectious diseases, 5, 19, 21, 24, 60, 90, 134, 148

influenza, 4, 18, 34, 88, 91, 108

interstitial lung disease, 112

intestine, large, 60, 63, 158, 159, 162, 164–65, 167, 168, 170

intestine, small, 26, 158, 159, 164, 167

intracranial pressure, 187–88, 200–201

intravenous immunoglobulin, 80

intravenous procedural sedation, 81

Introduction to the Study of Experimental Medicine (Bernard), 198

iris, 117–19, 147

Ixodes tick, 82

Jack-in-the-Box restaurant, 64, 65

Jamaica Plain, Massachusetts, 139

Jamestown, Virgina, 123

jejunum, 159

jimsonweed, 123

Johns Hopkins Hospital (Baltimore), 20, 153

Jones, Samuel, 138

Journal of the American Medical Association (JAMA), 51, 110

Kakamega, Kenya, 10

Karmali, Mohamed, 64, 69

Kentucky Lake, 40

keratitis, 51

Kern, David, 112–14

Kerner, Justin, 6–8, 11

kidney failure, 61–62, 82

Kim, Melanie, 66

Kingston, New York, 3

Koch, Robert, 7, 28, 38, 153–55

Kowalski, Robert, 167

L.L. Bean, 114

Lancet, The, 108, 124, 177

Landry de Thézillat, Jean-Baptiste Octave, 78

Lands End, 114

latent period, 108

Legionnaire's disease, 98

Lenin, Vladimir, 205

Lett, Susan, 66–67, 69, 70–71, 114, 204–5

leukemia, 53, 90, 145

Levy, Don, 166, 168

Lind, James, 202

liver disease, 164, 171–72, 177–79

Loch Maree, Scotland, 8

loofah, 53–57

Louis-Napoléon (emperor of France), 198

low-density lipoproteins (LDL), 167

lumbar puncture. *See* spinal tap

lung cancer, 91

Lyme disease, 34, 48, 80, 82–83, 193

lymph nodes, 43, 49, 88

lymphocytes, 90, 144–45, 150

Macbeth, 123, 124

McCollum, Elmer, 203

McDonald's, 63–64

macule, 48

magnetic resonance angiography (MRA), 77

magnetic resonance imaging (MRI), 77, 86, 87, 188–91

malaria, 34, 109, 144

Malden Mills, 103–4, 106, 108, 110–12, 114–15

malignant tumor, 100, 147, 175

Mallon, Mary. *See* Typhoid Mary

mania, 124

Massachusetts Department of Public Health, 204, 208

Massachusetts Environmental Protection Agency, 98

optic nerve fenestration, 196
oral rehydration. *See* rehydration
therapy
orange juice, 27, 32, 34
oxygen, absence of. *See* anaerobic
oxygen-free environment, 11, 16
oxygen therapy, 112
Oyster Bay, Long Island, 28, 29
ozone, 107

PA. See *Pseudomonas aeruginosa*
papilledema, 186–88, 191–92, 195
papule, 48–49, 56
paralysis, 7, 11, 12, 78–80, 83–87
paralytic fish poisoning, 43
Parana River, 23
parasympathetic autonomic nervous
system, 118
parathyroid gland, 152, 201
parathyroid hormone (PTH), 201, 205
Paré, Ambrose, 161–62
Parthian Wars, 123
Pasteur, Louis, 93
pasteurized, 69
Patagonia, 114
Pawtucket, Rhode Island, 112–13
pediatricians, 34, 58, 66, 131, 179, 197
pediatric neurosurgeon, 117, 121
peritoneal cavity. *See* abdominal cavity
peritoneum, 159–60, 171–72
persimmon, 164
Peter Bent Brigham Hospital
(Boston), 95
Peters, John, 105, 106–7, 109–10, 112
pharmacobezoar, 164
phytobezoars, 163, 168
Pickering, Great Britain, 23
piranhas, 41–42, 44
plague, 124, 161, 163, 169
plant fiber, 168
plasma cells, 90

plasma exchange, 80
plasmapheresis, 81–82, 85
Plesiomonas shigelloides (PS), 36–37,
38–40, 41, 42, 44
Plunkett, Roy, 107–8
Plutarch, 123
pneumonia, 19, 20, 52, 88, 90–91, 95,
97, 100, 116
pneumonitis. *See* pneumonia
Polarfleece, Polartec, 114
polymer, 107, 109–11, 114–15
polymer-fume fever, 107–15
polymorphonuclear leukocytes, 90
polytetrafluoroethylene (PTFE), 107–
8, 109, 110, 111, 114
pomace, 69
Posner, Jill, 81–83, 86
posterior fossa, 188
post-operative period, 168
post-renal, 61
potassium sorbate, 70
potato, 9, 122
Potissier (doctor who described
metal-fume fever), 109
precipitin test, 97–99
pre-renal, 61
Priniciples and Practice of Medicine
(Osler), 20
Pseudomonas aeruginosa, 49–50
Pseudomonas folliculitis, 52
pseudotumor cerebri, 191–93, 195–
96
psyllium husk, 164
PTFE (polytetrafluoroethylene), 107–
8, 109, 110, 111, 114
public health, 21–22, 25, 32, 38, 44, 63,
66, 70, 97, 99, 100, 105, 131, 135, 137,
203, 204, 208
pupils, 6, 116–22, 124–28, 154, 186
pupillary size, 118
pustule (papule), 48–49

putrefaction, 93

putrescine, 136, 139

pyocyanin, 50, 54

pyoverdin, 50, 54

Quincke, Heinrich, 191–92

rabies, 97, 124

Ramsey, Jesse, 34, 36–38, 45

raquiferol, 206

Reed, Walter, 21

rehydration therapy, 35, 60

renal failure, 61–62, 65

reportable disease, 40

respiratory system, 34, 110

retina, 118–19, 187–88, 190

retinol. *See* vitamin A

retinol activity equivalents (RAE), 194

rickets, 202–3, 209

Riley, Lee, 63

Riverside Hospital (New York), 30–31

Rockford, Illinois, 71

rocky mountain spotted fever, 83–84

rose spots, 20

rotavirus, 36

Rubin, Robert H., 90–97, 112, 114

ruminating, 161

salmonella, 20, 41, 60

Salmonella typhi, 20, 22–24, 27–28

Salt Lake City-County Health Department, 52

salt tolerant, 141

Sands Point, Long Island, 29

sanitation, 21, 25

sausage poisoning, 6, 7

schistosomiasis, 80

Scombridae, 135

scombroid poisoning, 43, 135–37, 139–43

scopolamine, 122, 127

Seiferth, John, 137–39

sepsis, 43, 144

serotype, 55, 63, 66

serum calcium, 198, 200

Setnik, Gary, 116–21, 127

sexually transmitted diseases, 49

Shakespeare, William, 124

shelf life, 141

shellfish, 21, 38–40, 43, 135

Sherwood, R. J., 111

shigella, 36, 60

shingles, 48–49

shunt procedure, 179

sick building syndrome, 99

silicosis, 92

sodium benzoate, 70

Solanacea, 122–23

Soper, George, 28–31

Spanish-American War, 21, 32, 122, 161

spinal canal, 190

spinal tap, 12, 40, 79, 80–82, 86, 87, 103, 120, 190–92, 196

sponges, 53–54, 55–57

spontaneous generation of life, 94

spores, 8, 9, 11, 14, 16, 91, 94

strep tonsillitis, 35

Strohl, André, 79

stroke, 4, 14, 31, 76–78, 153, 191

Stubblefield, Phil, 131, 133–34, 136–37

subarachnoid hemorrhage, 120–21

subarachnoid space, 120, 191, 195

sulfur dioxide, 107

Sullivan County Public Health Nursing Services, 25

Summerton, New York, 18

swimming pool, 43, 50, 52, 56, 132

swimming pool granuloma, 43

swine-flu immunization, 80

sympathetic autonomic nervous system, 118

syphilis, 35, 79, 145, 148